2. Quinoa salad with spinach, chickpeas, and lemon vinaigrette

Ingredients:
- 1 cup quinoa, rinsed
- 2 cups water or vegetable broth
- 1 can (15 ounces) chickpeas, drained and rinsed
- 2 cups fresh spinach leaves, chopped
- 1/2 red onion, finely chopped
- 1/2 cup cherry tomatoes, halved
- 1/4 cup chopped fresh parsley
- 1/4 cup crumbled feta cheese (optional)
- Salt and pepper to taste

Lemon Vinaigrette:
- 1/4 cup extra virgin olive oil
- Zest and juice of 1 lemon
- 1 tablespoon honey or maple syrup
- 1 clove garlic, minced
- 1 teaspoon Dijon mustard
- Salt and pepper to taste

Instructions:

1. In a medium saucepan, combine quinoa and water or vegetable broth. Bring to a boil, then reduce heat to low, cover, and simmer for about 15 minutes, or until quinoa is cooked and water is absorbed. Remove from heat and let it cool slightly.

2. In a large mixing bowl, combine cooked quinoa, chickpeas, chopped spinach, red onion, cherry tomatoes, and chopped parsley. Toss to combine.

3. In a small bowl, whisk together the ingredients for the lemon vinaigrette: olive oil, lemon zest, lemon juice, honey or maple syrup, minced garlic, Dijon mustard, salt, and pepper.

4. Pour the lemon vinaigrette over the quinoa salad and toss until everything is evenly coated.

5. If using, sprinkle crumbled feta cheese over the salad.

6. Season with additional salt and pepper to taste, if needed.

7. Serve the quinoa salad immediately, or refrigerate for at least 30 minutes to allow the flavors to meld before serving.

3. Turkey and vegetable soup

Ingredients:
- 1 pound ground turkey
- 2 tablespoons olive oil
- 1 large onion, chopped
- 3 cloves garlic, minced
- 2 carrots, peeled and sliced
- 2 celery stalks, sliced
- 1 red bell pepper, chopped
- 1 zucchini, chopped
- 1 can (14.5 ounces) diced tomatoes
- 6 cups low-sodium chicken or vegetable broth
- 1 teaspoon dried thyme
- 1 teaspoon dried oregano
- 1 teaspoon dried basil
- 1 bay leaf
- Salt and pepper to taste
- 2 cups fresh spinach or kale, chopped
- Fresh parsley, chopped (for garnish)

Instructions:

1. In a large pot, heat olive oil over medium heat. Add the ground turkey and cook until browned, breaking it up into small pieces as it cooks. Season with a pinch of salt and pepper. Once cooked through, remove the turkey from the pot and set aside.

2. In the same pot, add the chopped onion, garlic, carrots, and celery. Cook for about 5-7 minutes, until the vegetables start to soften.

3. Add the red bell pepper and zucchini to the pot, and cook for another 3-4 minutes.

4. Stir in the diced tomatoes (with their juices) and return the cooked ground turkey to the pot.

5. Pour in the chicken or vegetable broth and add the dried thyme, oregano, basil, bay leaf, and additional salt and pepper to taste. Bring the soup to a boil, then reduce the heat to low and let it simmer for about 20-25 minutes, until the vegetables are tender.

6. Add the chopped spinach or kale to the pot and simmer for an additional 5 minutes, until the greens are wilted.

7. Remove the bay leaf and taste the soup, adjusting the seasoning if necessary. Serve hot, garnished with fresh chopped parsley if desired.

Introduction

Welcome to **_"Cookbook For Arthritis Weight Loss: Arthritis-Friendly Recipes for a Healthy Weight"_**. This book is designed to be your trusted companion in the journey towards better joint health and weight management. Whether you've been living with arthritis for years or have recently been diagnosed, finding the right balance between nourishing your body and maintaining a healthy weight can significantly impact your quality of life.

Arthritis is a condition characterized by inflammation and pain in the joints, often exacerbated by excess weight, which puts additional strain on already stressed joints. Managing your weight can play a crucial role in reducing symptoms, improving mobility, and enhancing overall well-being. However, achieving and maintaining a healthy weight while ensuring proper nutrition requires a thoughtful approach, especially when dealing with arthritis.

This book is here to guide you through that process. We have carefully curated a collection of delicious, nutritious, and arthritis-friendly recipes that support weight loss and joint health. Each recipe is crafted to provide essential nutrients, reduce inflammation, and promote a healthy weight, all while being easy to prepare and enjoyable to eat.

In addition to the recipes, we've included valuable information on the connection between diet, weight, and arthritis. You'll find insights into how certain foods can help manage inflammation, the importance of balanced nutrition, and practical strategies for weight loss tailored to those with arthritis. We've also provided tips on portion control, meal planning, and mindful eating to support your journey.

Here's what you can expect from this book:
- **_Nutrient-Rich Recipes:_** Discover a variety of dishes that are not only tasty but also packed with vitamins, minerals, and anti-inflammatory ingredients. From energizing breakfasts to satisfying dinners and snacks, each recipe is designed to support your weight loss goals and joint health.

- **_Practical Tips and Strategies:_** Learn effective weight loss strategies that are gentle on your joints, including low-impact exercises, stress management techniques, and tips for staying motivated.

- **_Meal Planning Guidance:_** Find helpful advice on planning your meals, grocery shopping, and stocking your kitchen with arthritis-friendly and weight loss-promoting ingredients.

- **_Scientific Insights:_** Gain a better understanding of how diet and weight influence arthritis symptoms, with easy-to-digest explanations of current research.

1. Grilled salmon with roasted vegetables

Ingredients:
- 2 salmon fillets
- 2 tablespoons olive oil
- 2 cloves garlic, minced
- 1 teaspoon dried thyme
- Salt and pepper to taste
- 2 cups mixed vegetables (such as bell peppers, zucchini, and carrots), chopped
- 1 tablespoon balsamic vinegar
- 1 tablespoon honey
- Fresh parsley for garnish (optional)

Instructions:
1. Preheat your grill to medium-high heat.

2. In a small bowl, mix together olive oil, minced garlic, dried thyme, salt, and pepper.

3. Brush the salmon fillets with the olive oil mixture on both sides.

4. Place the salmon fillets on the grill and cook for about 4-5 minutes on each side, or until the salmon is cooked through and flakes easily with a fork.

5. While the salmon is grilling, prepare the vegetables. Toss the chopped vegetables with olive oil, salt, and pepper.

6. Spread the vegetables out on a baking sheet lined with parchment paper and roast in the oven at 400°F (200°C) for about 20-25 minutes, or until they are tender and slightly caramelized.

7. In a small bowl, whisk together balsamic vinegar and honey.

8. Drizzle the balsamic-honey mixture over the roasted vegetables and toss to coat.

9. Once the salmon is done, serve it hot alongside the roasted vegetables.

10. Garnish with fresh parsley if desired.

Enjoy your delicious and arthritis-friendly grilled salmon with roasted vegetables!

4. Baked sweet potato with Greek yogurt and cinnamon

Ingredients:
- 2 medium sweet potatoes
- 1/2 cup Greek yogurt
- 1-2 tablespoons honey (optional)
- 1/2 teaspoon ground cinnamon
- Pinch of salt
- Fresh mint leaves (optional, for garnish)

Instructions:
1. Preheat your oven to 400°F (200°C).

2. Wash the sweet potatoes and pat them dry with a paper towel.

3. Pierce the sweet potatoes several times with a fork to allow steam to escape during baking.

4. Place the sweet potatoes on a baking sheet lined with parchment paper or aluminum foil.

5. Bake the sweet potatoes in the preheated oven for 45-60 minutes, or until they are tender when pierced with a fork.

6. While the sweet potatoes are baking, prepare the Greek yogurt topping. In a small bowl, mix together the Greek yogurt, honey (if using), ground cinnamon, and a pinch of salt. Adjust sweetness to your taste.

7. Once the sweet potatoes are baked and tender, remove them from the oven and let them cool slightly.

8. Slice each sweet potato lengthwise down the center, without cutting all the way through.

9. Gently press the ends of the sweet potatoes together to open up the center.

10. Spoon the Greek yogurt mixture over the center of each sweet potato.

11. Garnish with fresh mint leaves, if desired.

12. Serve immediately while the sweet potatoes are warm.

Enjoy this delightful and nutritious baked sweet potato topped with creamy Greek yogurt and fragrant cinnamon!

5. Zucchini noodles with tomato and basil sauce

Ingredients:
- 4 medium zucchini
- 2 tablespoons olive oil
- 3 cloves garlic, minced
- 1 can (14.5 ounces) diced tomatoes
- 1/4 teaspoon red pepper flakes (optional, for a spicy kick)
- Salt and pepper to taste
- 1/4 cup chopped fresh basil leaves
- Grated Parmesan cheese for garnish (optional)

Instructions:
1. Using a spiralizer or vegetable peeler, spiralize or julienne the zucchini into noodles. Set aside.

2. In a large skillet, heat olive oil over medium heat. Add the minced garlic and sauté for about 1 minute, until fragrant.

3. Add the diced tomatoes (with their juices) to the skillet. If you like a bit of heat, you can also add the red pepper flakes at this stage.

4. Season the tomato sauce with salt and pepper to taste. Allow the sauce to simmer for about 10-15 minutes, stirring occasionally, until it thickens slightly.

5. Once the sauce has thickened, add the zucchini noodles to the skillet. Toss the noodles with the sauce until they are well coated.

6. Cook the zucchini noodles for 2-3 minutes, stirring occasionally, until they are just tender but still have a slight crunch. Be careful not to overcook, as zucchini noodles can become mushy if cooked for too long.

7. Remove the skillet from heat and stir in the chopped fresh basil.

8. Taste and adjust the seasoning if necessary.

9. Serve the zucchini noodles with tomato and basil sauce immediately, garnished with grated Parmesan cheese if desired.

Enjoy this light and flavorful dish of zucchini noodles with tomato and basil sauce! It's perfect for a quick and healthy weeknight meal.

6. Grilled chicken with mango salsa

Ingredients:
- 4 boneless, skinless chicken breasts
- 2 tablespoons olive oil
- 1 teaspoon paprika
- 1 teaspoon garlic powder
- 1 teaspoon onion powder
- Salt and pepper to taste

For the Mango Salsa:
- 2 ripe mangoes, peeled, pitted, and diced
- 1/2 red onion, finely chopped
- 1 red bell pepper, diced
- 1 jalapeño pepper, seeded and minced (optional, for heat)
- Juice of 1 lime
- 2 tablespoons chopped fresh cilantro
- Salt and pepper to taste

Instructions:
1. Preheat your grill to medium-high heat.

2. In a small bowl, mix together olive oil, paprika, garlic powder, onion powder, salt, and pepper to create a marinade.

3. Place the chicken breasts in a shallow dish or resealable plastic bag, and pour the marinade over them. Make sure the chicken is evenly coated. Let it marinate in the refrigerator for at least 30 minutes, or up to 4 hours.

4. While the chicken is marinating, prepare the mango salsa. In a medium bowl, combine diced mangoes, chopped red onion, diced red bell pepper, minced jalapeño pepper (if using), lime juice, chopped cilantro, salt, and pepper. Mix well and set aside.

5. Once the chicken has finished marinating, remove it from the refrigerator and let it sit at room temperature for about 10 minutes.

6. Grill the chicken breasts for about 6-8 minutes per side, or until they are cooked through and reach an internal temperature of 165°F (75°C). Cooking time may vary depending on the thickness of the chicken breasts.

7. Once the chicken is cooked, remove it from the grill and let it rest for a few minutes before serving. Serve the grilled chicken breasts hot, topped with mango salsa

7. Lentil and sweet potato curry

Ingredients:

- 1 cup dry lentils (green or brown), rinsed and drained
- 2 medium sweet potatoes, peeled and diced
- 1 onion, chopped
- 3 cloves garlic, minced
- 1 tablespoon ginger, minced
- 1 can (14 ounces) diced tomatoes
- 1 can (14 ounces) coconut milk
- 2 cups vegetable broth or water
- 2 tablespoons curry powder
- 1 teaspoon ground cumin
- 1 teaspoon ground turmeric
- 1/2 teaspoon ground coriander
- 1/4 teaspoon cayenne pepper (optional, for heat)
- Salt and pepper to taste
- 2 tablespoons olive oil
- Fresh cilantro, chopped (for garnish)
- Cooked rice or naan bread (for serving)

Instructions:

1. In a large pot or Dutch oven, heat olive oil over medium heat. Add the chopped onion and cook for 3-4 minutes until softened.

2. Add the minced garlic and ginger to the pot, and cook for another 1-2 minutes until fragrant.

3. Stir in the curry powder, ground cumin, ground turmeric, ground coriander, and cayenne pepper (if using). Cook the spices for about 1 minute to toast them and release their flavors.
4. Add the diced sweet potatoes, rinsed lentils, diced tomatoes (with their juices), coconut milk, and vegetable broth or water to the pot. Stir well to combine.

5. Bring the mixture to a boil, then reduce the heat to low and cover the pot. Let the curry simmer for about 20-25 minutes, or until the lentils and sweet potatoes are tender, stirring occasionally.

6. Once the lentils and sweet potatoes are cooked through, season the curry with salt and pepper to taste. Adjust the seasoning and consistency of the curry by adding more broth or water if needed.

7. Serve the lentil and sweet potato curry hot, garnished with chopped fresh cilantro. Enjoy with cooked rice or naan bread.

This lentil and sweet potato curry is a satisfying and wholesome meal that's perfect for chilly evenings. Feel free to customize it with your favorite vegetables or additional spices according to your taste preferences.

8. Spinach and feta stuffed chicken breasts

Ingredients:
- 4 boneless, skinless chicken breasts
- 2 cups fresh spinach leaves, chopped
- 1/2 cup crumbled feta cheese
- 2 cloves garlic, minced
- 1 tablespoon olive oil
- 1 teaspoon dried oregano
- 1 teaspoon dried basil
- Salt and pepper to taste
- Toothpicks or kitchen twine (for securing)

Instructions:

1. Preheat your oven to 375°F (190°C).

2. In a skillet, heat olive oil over medium heat. Add minced garlic and sauté for about 1 minute until fragrant.

3. Add chopped spinach to the skillet and cook until wilted, about 2-3 minutes. Remove from heat and let it cool slightly.

4. In a mixing bowl, combine the cooked spinach with crumbled feta cheese, dried oregano, dried basil, salt, and pepper. Mix well to combine.

5. Use a sharp knife to make a horizontal slit along the side of each chicken breast to create a pocket, being careful not to cut all the way through.

6. Stuff each chicken breast with the spinach and feta mixture, dividing it evenly among them. Secure the openings with toothpicks or kitchen twine to keep the filling from falling out.

7. Season the outside of the chicken breasts with salt, pepper, and a drizzle of olive oil.

8. Heat an oven-safe skillet or baking dish over medium-high heat. Once hot, add the stuffed chicken breasts to the skillet and sear for 2-3 minutes on each side until golden brown.

9. Transfer the skillet or baking dish to the preheated oven and bake for 20-25 minutes, or until the chicken is cooked through and no longer pink in the center, with an internal temperature of 165°F (75°C).

10. Once cooked, remove the stuffed chicken breasts from the oven and let them rest for a few minutes before serving.

11. Remove the toothpicks or kitchen twine before serving. Serve the spinach and feta stuffed chicken breasts hot, garnished with fresh herbs if desired

9. Tuna salad lettuce wraps

Ingredients:
- 2 cans (5 ounces each) tuna, drained
- 1/4 cup mayonnaise or Greek yogurt
- 2 tablespoons Dijon mustard
- 2 tablespoons finely chopped red onion
- 2 tablespoons finely chopped celery
- 1 tablespoon lemon juice
- 1/4 teaspoon garlic powder
- Salt and pepper to taste
- 8 large lettuce leaves (such as romaine or butter lettuce)
- Sliced cucumber, avocado, or tomato (optional, for topping)
- Fresh parsley or dill, chopped (for garnish)

Instructions:
1. In a mixing bowl, combine drained tuna, mayonnaise or Greek yogurt, Dijon mustard, chopped red onion, chopped celery, lemon juice, garlic powder, salt, and pepper. Mix well until all ingredients are evenly combined.

2. Taste the tuna salad and adjust the seasoning if necessary.

3. Lay out the lettuce leaves on a clean work surface.

4. Spoon the tuna salad mixture onto each lettuce leaf, dividing it evenly among them.

5. If desired, top each lettuce wrap with sliced cucumber, avocado, or tomato for extra flavor and texture.

6. Garnish the lettuce wraps with chopped fresh parsley or dill for a burst of freshness.

7. Carefully roll up each lettuce leaf to enclose the tuna salad filling, similar to a burrito or wrap.

8. Secure the wraps with toothpicks if needed to hold them together.

9. Serve the tuna salad lettuce wraps immediately, or refrigerate them for later.

Enjoy these light and flavorful tuna salad lettuce wraps as a nutritious and satisfying meal or snack! They're perfect for a low-carb or gluten-free diet.

10. Cauliflower rice stir-fry with vegetables and tofu

Ingredients:
- 1 head cauliflower
- 1 block firm tofu, pressed and cubed
- 2 tablespoons soy sauce or tamari
- 1 tablespoon sesame oil
- 2 tablespoons olive oil or vegetable oil, divided
- 2 cloves garlic, minced
- 1 tablespoon fresh ginger, minced
- 1 onion, thinly sliced
- 2 carrots, julienned

- 1 bell pepper, thinly sliced
- 1 cup broccoli florets
- 1 cup snap peas, trimmed
- 2 green onions, chopped (for garnish)
- Sesame seeds (for garnish)
- Salt and pepper to taste

For the Stir-Fry Sauce:
- 3 tablespoons soy sauce or tamari
- 1 tablespoon rice vinegar
- 1 tablespoon honey or maple syrup
- 1 teaspoon sesame oil
- 1 teaspoon cornstarch
- 1/4 cup water

Instructions:
1. Remove the leaves and core from the cauliflower and cut it into florets. Working in batches, pulse the cauliflower florets in a food processor until they resemble rice grains. Alternatively, you can use a box grater to grate the cauliflower. Set the cauliflower rice aside.

2. In a small bowl, whisk together the ingredients for the stir-fry sauce: soy sauce or tamari, rice vinegar, honey or maple syrup, sesame oil, cornstarch, and water. Set aside.

3. Heat 1 tablespoon of olive oil or vegetable oil in a large skillet or wok over medium-high heat. Add the cubed tofu and cook until golden brown on all sides, about 5-7 minutes. Remove the tofu from the skillet and set aside.

4. In the same skillet, add another tablespoon of oil if needed. Add minced garlic and ginger, and sauté for about 1 minute until fragrant. Add sliced onion, julienned carrots, sliced bell pepper, broccoli florets, and snap peas to the skillet. Stir-fry the vegetables for about 5-7 minutes until they are tender-crisp.

5. Push the vegetables to one side of the skillet and add the cauliflower rice to the empty side. Stir-fry the cauliflower rice for about 3-4 minutes until it is heated through and slightly tender. Return the cooked tofu to the skillet with the vegetables and cauliflower rice.

6. Pour the stir-fry sauce over the tofu, vegetables, and cauliflower rice. Stir well to coat everything evenly with the sauce. Cook for another 2-3 minutes until the sauce has thickened slightly and everything is heated through. Taste and adjust the seasoning with salt and pepper if needed.

7. Remove the skillet from heat and garnish the cauliflower rice stir-fry with chopped green onions and sesame seeds. Serve hot and enjoy your cauliflower rice stir-fry with vegetables and tofu!

11. Baked cod with olive oil and herbs

Ingredients:
- 4 cod fillets (about 6 ounces each)
- 2 tablespoons extra virgin olive oil
- 2 cloves garlic, minced
- 1 tablespoon fresh lemon juice
- 1 teaspoon dried oregano
- 1 teaspoon dried thyme
- Salt and pepper to taste
- Lemon wedges for serving
- Chopped fresh parsley for garnish

Instructions:

1. Preheat your oven to 400°F (200°C). Lightly grease a baking dish with olive oil or cooking spray.

2. Pat the cod fillets dry with paper towels and place them in the prepared baking dish.

3. In a small bowl, whisk together the extra virgin olive oil, minced garlic, fresh lemon juice, dried oregano, dried thyme, salt, and pepper.

4. Drizzle the olive oil and herb mixture over the cod fillets, making sure to coat them evenly.

5. Bake the cod in the preheated oven for 12-15 minutes, or until the fish is opaque and flakes easily with a fork.

6. If desired, you can broil the cod for an additional 1-2 minutes at the end to brown the top slightly.

7. Remove the baked cod from the oven and let it rest for a few minutes.

8. Serve the cod hot, garnished with chopped fresh parsley and lemon wedges on the side for squeezing over the fish.

Enjoy this delicious and healthy baked cod with olive oil and herbs! It pairs well with a variety of side dishes such as steamed vegetables, roasted potatoes, or a fresh salad.

12. Quinoa and black bean burrito bowls

Ingredients:
- 1 cup quinoa, rinsed
- 2 cups water or vegetable broth
- 1 can (15 ounces) black beans, drained and rinsed
- 1 tablespoon olive oil
- 1 onion, diced
- 2 cloves garlic, minced
- 1 bell pepper, diced
- 1 teaspoon ground cumin
- 1 teaspoon chili powder
- Salt and pepper to taste
- Juice of 1 lime
- 1 avocado, sliced
- Fresh cilantro, chopped (for garnish)
- Sour cream or Greek yogurt (optional, for serving)
- Salsa or pico de gallo (optional, for serving)

Instructions:

1. In a medium saucepan, combine quinoa and water or vegetable broth. Bring to a boil, then reduce heat to low, cover, and simmer for about 15-20 minutes, or until quinoa is cooked and water is absorbed. Remove from heat and fluff with a fork.

2. While the quinoa is cooking, heat olive oil in a skillet over medium heat. Add diced onion and cook for 2-3 minutes until softened.

3. Add minced garlic and diced bell pepper to the skillet, and cook for another 2-3 minutes until the vegetables are tender.

4. Stir in the drained and rinsed black beans, ground cumin, chili powder, salt, and pepper. Cook for a few more minutes until the beans are heated through and the flavors are combined.

5. Once the quinoa is cooked, remove it from the heat and stir in the lime juice.

6. To assemble the burrito bowls, divide the cooked quinoa among serving bowls. Top each bowl with the black bean and vegetable mixture.

7. Add sliced avocado on top of each bowl, and garnish with chopped fresh cilantro.

8. Serve the quinoa and black bean burrito bowls with optional toppings such as sour cream or Greek yogurt, and salsa or pico de gallo on the side.

Enjoy these flavorful and customizable quinoa and black bean burrito bowls for a wholesome and delicious meal! They're packed with protein, fiber, and plenty of fresh ingredients.

13. Stuffed bell peppers with ground turkey and brown rice

Ingredients:
- 1 cup tomato sauce or marinara sauce
- 1 teaspoon dried oregano
- 1 teaspoon dried basil
- Salt and pepper to taste
- 1 cup shredded mozzarella cheese (optional)
- Fresh parsley or basil, chopped (for garnish)
- 4 large bell peppers (any color), halved and seeds removed
- 1 pound lean ground turkey
- 1 cup cooked brown rice
- 1 onion, finely chopped
- 2 cloves garlic, minced
- 1 can (14.5 ounces) diced tomatoes, drained

Instructions:

1. Preheat your oven to 375°F (190°C). Lightly grease a baking dish large enough to hold the bell pepper halves.

2. In a large skillet, cook the ground turkey over medium heat until browned and cooked through, breaking it up with a spoon as it cooks.

3. Add chopped onion and minced garlic to the skillet with the cooked turkey. Cook for 3-4 minutes until the onion is softened and translucent.

4. Stir in the cooked brown rice, diced tomatoes, tomato sauce, dried oregano, dried basil, salt, and pepper. Cook for another 2-3 minutes until everything is well combined and heated through.

5. Taste the filling and adjust the seasoning if needed. Place the halved bell peppers in the prepared baking dish, cut side up.

6. Spoon the turkey and rice mixture evenly into each bell pepper half, pressing down gently to pack the filling. If desired, sprinkle shredded mozzarella cheese over the stuffed bell peppers.

7. Cover the baking dish with aluminum foil and bake in the preheated oven for 25-30 minutes, or until the bell peppers are tender.

8. Remove the foil and bake for an additional 5-10 minutes, or until the cheese is melted and bubbly.

9. Once cooked, remove the stuffed bell peppers from the oven and let them cool slightly before serving. Garnish with chopped fresh parsley or basil before serving.

Enjoy these delicious stuffed bell peppers with ground turkey and brown rice as a wholesome and satisfying meal! They're perfect for a family dinner or meal prep for the week ahead.

14. Roasted Brussels sprouts with balsamic glaze

Ingredients:
- 1 pound Brussels sprouts, trimmed and halved
- 2 tablespoons olive oil
- Salt and pepper to taste
- 2 tablespoons balsamic vinegar
- 1 tablespoon honey or maple syrup (optional, for added sweetness)
- 1-2 cloves garlic, minced (optional, for added flavor)
- Fresh thyme leaves or chopped parsley for garnish (optional)

Instructions:
1. Preheat your oven to 400°F (200°C) and line a baking sheet with parchment paper or aluminum foil.

2. In a large mixing bowl, toss the halved Brussels sprouts with olive oil until evenly coated.

3. Season the Brussels sprouts with salt and pepper to taste, and toss again to distribute the seasoning.

4. Arrange the Brussels sprouts in a single layer on the prepared baking sheet, cut side down.

5. Roast the Brussels sprouts in the preheated oven for 20-25 minutes, or until they are tender and golden brown, stirring halfway through the cooking time for even browning.

6. While the Brussels sprouts are roasting, prepare the balsamic glaze. In a small saucepan, combine balsamic vinegar, honey or maple syrup (if using), and minced garlic (if using). Bring the mixture to a simmer over medium heat, then reduce the heat to low and cook for 5-7 minutes, stirring occasionally, until the glaze has thickened slightly.

7. Once the Brussels sprouts are done roasting, transfer them to a serving dish. Drizzle the balsamic glaze over the roasted Brussels sprouts, using as much or as little as desired.

8. Garnish with fresh thyme leaves or chopped parsley, if using. Serve the roasted Brussels sprouts with balsamic glaze immediately as a delicious side dish.

Enjoy the sweet and tangy flavor of these roasted Brussels sprouts with balsamic glaze! They're perfect for serving alongside roasted meats, grilled chicken, or as part of a vegetarian meal.

15. Grilled portobello mushroom caps with avocado salsa

Ingredients:
- 4 large portobello mushroom caps, stems removed
- 2 tablespoons olive oil
- 2 cloves garlic, minced
- Salt and pepper to taste

- 1 small tomato, diced
- 1/4 cup red onion, finely chopped
- 1 jalapeño pepper, seeded and finely chopped
- Juice of 1 lime
- 2 tablespoons chopped fresh cilantro
- Salt and pepper to taste

For the Avocado Salsa:
- 2 ripe avocados, diced

Instructions:
1. Preheat your grill to medium-high heat.

2. In a small bowl, whisk together the olive oil, minced garlic, salt, and pepper.

3. Brush both sides of the portobello mushroom caps with the olive oil mixture.

4. Place the mushroom caps on the preheated grill, gill side down, and cook for about 4-5 minutes.

5. Flip the mushroom caps and continue to grill for an additional 4-5 minutes, or until they are tender and grill marks appear.

6. While the mushroom caps are grilling, prepare the avocado salsa. In a medium bowl, combine diced avocados, diced tomato, chopped red onion, chopped jalapeño pepper, lime juice, chopped cilantro, salt, and pepper. Gently toss to combine.

7. Once the mushroom caps are grilled to your liking, remove them from the grill and let them cool slightly.

8. To serve, place the grilled portobello mushroom caps on a serving platter or individual plates. Spoon the avocado salsa over the grilled mushroom caps.

9. Garnish with additional cilantro if desired. Serve the grilled portobello mushroom caps with avocado salsa immediately.

Enjoy these flavorful and nutritious grilled portobello mushroom caps with avocado salsa as a light meal or appetizer! They're perfect for summer grilling and bursting with fresh flavors.

16. Lentil and vegetable soup

Ingredients:
- 1 cup dried lentils (green or brown), rinsed and drained
- 6 cups vegetable broth
- 2 tablespoons olive oil
- 1 onion, diced
- 2 carrots, peeled and diced
- 2 celery stalks, diced
- 2 cloves garlic, minced
- 1 can (14.5 ounces) diced tomatoes
- 1 teaspoon dried thyme
- 1 teaspoon dried oregano
- 1 bay leaf
- Salt and pepper to taste
- 2 cups chopped fresh spinach or kale
- Fresh parsley, chopped (for garnish)
- Lemon wedges (optional, for serving)

Instructions:
1. In a large pot, heat olive oil over medium heat. Add diced onion, carrots, and celery. Cook for about 5-7 minutes, until the vegetables are softened.

2. Add minced garlic to the pot and cook for an additional 1-2 minutes, until fragrant.

3. Stir in the rinsed lentils, diced tomatoes (with their juices), vegetable broth, dried thyme, dried oregano, bay leaf, salt, and pepper.

4. Bring the soup to a boil, then reduce the heat to low and let it simmer, partially covered, for about 25-30 minutes, or until the lentils are tender.

5. Once the lentils are cooked, stir in the chopped fresh spinach or kale and cook for another 3-5 minutes until the greens are wilted.

6. Taste the soup and adjust the seasoning with salt and pepper if needed. Remove the bay leaf from the soup before serving.

7. Ladle the lentil and vegetable soup into bowls and garnish with chopped fresh parsley. Serve hot, optionally with lemon wedges on the side for squeezing over the soup.

Enjoy this wholesome and flavorful lentil and vegetable soup! It's perfect for a cozy dinner or meal prep for a week of nutritious lunches.

17. Baked salmon with pineapple salsa

Ingredients:
- 4 salmon fillets (about 6 ounces each)
- 2 tablespoons olive oil
- Salt and pepper to taste
- 2 cups diced pineapple
- 1/2 red bell pepper, diced
- 1/4 red onion, finely chopped
- 1 jalapeño pepper, seeded and minced
- Juice of 1 lime
- 2 tablespoons chopped fresh cilantro
- Pinch of salt
- Pinch of black pepper

Instructions:
1. Preheat your oven to 375°F (190°C).

2. Place the salmon fillets on a baking sheet lined with parchment paper or aluminum foil.

3. Drizzle the salmon fillets with olive oil and season with salt and pepper to taste.

4. Bake the salmon in the preheated oven for 12-15 minutes, or until the salmon is cooked through and flakes easily with a fork.

5. While the salmon is baking, prepare the pineapple salsa. In a medium bowl, combine diced pineapple, diced red bell pepper, finely chopped red onion, minced jalapeño pepper, lime juice, chopped cilantro, salt, and black pepper. Stir well to combine.

6. Once the salmon is done baking, remove it from the oven and let it cool slightly.

7. Serve the baked salmon hot, topped with the pineapple salsa.

8. Garnish with additional fresh cilantro if desired.

9. Serve immediately and enjoy your delicious baked salmon with pineapple salsa!

This dish pairs wonderfully with steamed rice or quinoa and a side of steamed vegetables for a complete meal. It's perfect for a weeknight dinner or for entertaining guests with its vibrant colors and flavors.

18. Vegetarian chili with sweet potatoes and black beans

Ingredients:
- 2 tablespoons olive oil
- 1 onion, diced
- 2 cloves garlic, minced
- 2 sweet potatoes, peeled and diced
- 1 bell pepper, diced
- 1 jalapeño pepper, seeded
and minced (optional, for heat)
- 1 can (15 ounces) black beans,
drained and rinsed
- 1 can (14.5 ounces) diced tomatoes
- 2 cups vegetable broth
- 1 tablespoon chili powder
- 1 teaspoon ground cumin
- 1 teaspoon smoked paprika
- Salt and pepper to taste
- Fresh cilantro, chopped (for garnish)
- Sour cream or Greek yogurt (optional, for serving)
- Avocado slices (optional, for serving)
- Lime wedges (optional, for serving)

Instructions:

1. Heat olive oil in a large pot or Dutch oven over medium heat.

2. Add diced onion to the pot and cook for 3-4 minutes until softened.

3. Stir in minced garlic and cook for another 1-2 minutes until fragrant.

4. Add diced sweet potatoes, diced bell pepper, and minced jalapeño pepper (if using) to the pot. Cook for about 5 minutes, stirring occasionally.

5. Stir in drained and rinsed black beans, diced tomatoes (with their juices), vegetable broth, chili powder, ground cumin, smoked paprika, salt, and pepper.

6. Bring the chili to a simmer, then reduce the heat to low and let it cook, partially covered, for about 20-25 minutes, or until the sweet potatoes are tender and the flavors have melded together, stirring occasionally.

7. Taste the chili and adjust the seasoning with salt and pepper if needed. Once the chili is done cooking, remove it from the heat. Serve the vegetarian chili hot, garnished with chopped fresh cilantro.

8. Optionally, serve with a dollop of sour cream or Greek yogurt, avocado slices, and lime wedges on the side for squeezing over the chili.

Enjoy this delicious and nutritious vegetarian chili with sweet potatoes and black beans! It's packed with protein, fiber, and plenty of flavor, making it a satisfying meal option for vegetarians and meat-lovers alike.

19. Grilled chicken with mango and avocado salad

Ingredients:

For the Grilled Chicken:
- 4 boneless, skinless chicken breasts
- 2 tablespoons olive oil
- 1 teaspoon paprika
- 1 teaspoon garlic powder
- 1 teaspoon onion powder
- Salt and pepper to taste

For the Mango and Avocado Salad:
- 2 ripe mangoes, peeled, pitted, and diced
- 2 ripe avocados, peeled, pitted, and diced
- 1/4 cup red onion, finely chopped
- 1/4 cup fresh cilantro, chopped
- Juice of 1 lime
- Salt and pepper to taste
- Mixed salad greens or spinach leaves

Instructions:

For the Grilled Chicken:

1. In a small bowl, mix together olive oil, paprika, garlic powder, onion powder, salt, and pepper to create a marinade.

2. Place the chicken breasts in a shallow dish or resealable plastic bag, and pour the marinade over them. Make sure the chicken is evenly coated. Let it marinate in the refrigerator for at least 30 minutes, or up to 4 hours.

3. Preheat your grill to medium-high heat. Remove the chicken breasts from the marinade and discard any excess marinade.

4. Grill the chicken breasts for about 6-8 minutes per side, or until they are cooked through and reach an internal temperature of 165°F (75°C). Cooking time may vary depending on the thickness of the chicken breasts.

5. Once cooked, remove the chicken breasts from the grill and let them rest for a few minutes before slicing.

For the Mango and Avocado Salad:

1. In a large bowl, combine diced mangoes, diced avocados, chopped red onion, chopped cilantro, and lime juice. Gently toss to combine. Season the salad with salt and pepper to taste.

2. Arrange mixed salad greens or spinach leaves on serving plates. Top the greens with the grilled chicken slices.

3. Spoon the mango and avocado salad over the grilled chicken. Garnish with additional cilantro if desired.

Enjoy this vibrant and flavorful grilled chicken with mango and avocado salad! It's a perfect balance of sweet and savory flavors, with a refreshing touch of citrus.

20. Quinoa and roasted vegetable salad

Ingredients:
- 1 cup quinoa, rinsed
- Assorted vegetables (e.g., bell peppers, zucchini, cherry tomatoes, red onion)
- 2 tablespoons olive oil
- Salt and pepper to taste
- 2 tablespoons balsamic vinegar
- 1 tablespoon honey or maple syrup (optional, for sweetness)
- 2 tablespoons chopped fresh basil or parsley

Instructions:
1. Preheat your oven to 400°F (200°C).

2. Toss assorted vegetables with olive oil, salt, and pepper on a baking sheet.

3. Roast in the preheated oven for 20-25 minutes, or until tender and slightly caramelized.

4. Meanwhile, cook quinoa according to package instructions and let it cool.

5. In a small bowl, whisk together balsamic vinegar and honey or maple syrup (if using).

6. In a large bowl, combine cooked quinoa, roasted vegetables, and balsamic dressing. Toss well to coat.

7. Garnish with chopped fresh basil or parsley before serving.

Enjoy this nutritious and flavorful quinoa and roasted vegetable salad! It's perfect as a side dish or a light meal on its own.

21. Baked tilapia with tomatoes and capers

Ingredients:
- 4 tilapia fillets
- 2 tablespoons olive oil
- Salt and pepper to taste
- 2 cups cherry tomatoes, halved
- 2 tablespoons capers, drained
- 2 cloves garlic, minced
- 1 tablespoon lemon juice
- 1 teaspoon dried oregano
- Fresh parsley, chopped (for garnish)

Instructions:

1. Preheat your oven to 400°F (200°C).

2. Place tilapia fillets in a baking dish and drizzle with olive oil. Season with salt and pepper.

3. In a bowl, mix together cherry tomatoes, capers, minced garlic, lemon juice, and dried oregano.

4. Spoon the tomato mixture over the tilapia fillets.

5. Bake in the preheated oven for 12-15 minutes, or until the tilapia is cooked through and flakes easily with a fork.

6. Garnish with chopped fresh parsley before serving.

Enjoy this simple and flavorful baked tilapia with tomatoes and capers! It's a light and delicious dish that's perfect for a quick weeknight dinner.

22. Turkey and vegetable lettuce wraps

Ingredients:
- 1 lb ground turkey
- 1 tablespoon olive oil
- 1 onion, finely chopped
- 2 cloves garlic, minced
- 1 red bell pepper, diced
- 1 zucchini, diced
- 1 carrot, shredded
- 1 teaspoon ground cumin
- 1 teaspoon chili powder
- Salt and pepper to taste
- 1/4 cup chopped fresh cilantro or parsley
- Iceberg or butter lettuce leaves, washed and dried

Instructions:

1. Heat olive oil in a large skillet over medium heat.

2. Add chopped onion and minced garlic to the skillet. Cook until softened and fragrant, about 2-3 minutes.

3. Add ground turkey to the skillet. Cook, breaking it apart with a spoon, until browned and cooked through.

4. Add diced bell pepper, diced zucchini, and shredded carrot to the skillet. Cook for another 5-7 minutes, until the vegetables are tender.

5. Season the mixture with ground cumin, chili powder, salt, and pepper. Stir well to combine.

6. Remove the skillet from the heat and stir in chopped fresh cilantro or parsley. Spoon the turkey and vegetable mixture onto lettuce leaves.

7. Roll up the lettuce leaves to form wraps. Serve immediately.

Enjoy these delicious and healthy turkey and vegetable lettuce wraps! They make a satisfying and nutritious meal or snack.

23. Lentil and spinach stuffed tomatoes

Ingredients:
- 4 large tomatoes
- 1 cup cooked lentils
- 1 cup fresh spinach, chopped
- 1 small onion, finely chopped
- 2 cloves garlic, minced
- 2 tablespoons olive oil
- 1 teaspoon dried oregano
- 1 teaspoon dried basil
- Salt and pepper to taste
- 1/4 cup grated Parmesan cheese (optional, for topping)

Instructions:
1. Preheat your oven to 375°F (190°C).

2. Cut the tops off the tomatoes and carefully scoop out the pulp and seeds using a spoon. Set the tomato shells aside.

3. Heat olive oil in a skillet over medium heat. Add chopped onion and minced garlic. Cook until softened and fragrant, about 2-3 minutes.

4. Add cooked lentils and chopped spinach to the skillet. Cook for another 2-3 minutes until the spinach wilts.

5. Stir in dried oregano, dried basil, salt, and pepper. Cook for an additional minute to combine the flavors.

6. Remove the skillet from the heat and let the mixture cool slightly.

7. Spoon the lentil and spinach mixture into the hollowed-out tomato shells, pressing down gently to pack the filling.

8. Place the stuffed tomatoes in a baking dish. If desired, sprinkle grated Parmesan cheese on top of each stuffed tomato.

9. Bake in the preheated oven for 20-25 minutes, or until the tomatoes are tender and the filling is heated through. Remove from the oven and let cool for a few minutes before serving.

Enjoy these flavorful lentil and spinach stuffed tomatoes as a delicious and nutritious appetizer or side dish! They're packed with protein, fiber, and vitamins.

24. Grilled asparagus with lemon and Parmesan

Ingredients:
- 1 bunch of asparagus, tough ends trimmed
- 2 tablespoons olive oil
- Zest of 1 lemon
- Juice of 1/2 lemon
- Salt and pepper to taste
- 1/4 cup grated Parmesan cheese

Instructions:
1. Preheat your grill to medium-high heat.

2. In a shallow dish, toss the trimmed asparagus spears with olive oil, lemon zest, lemon juice, salt, and pepper until evenly coated.

3. Place the asparagus spears on the preheated grill. Grill for 4-6 minutes, turning occasionally, until tender and slightly charred.

4. Remove the grilled asparagus from the grill and place them on a serving platter.

5. Sprinkle grated Parmesan cheese over the hot grilled asparagus.

6. Serve immediately.

Enjoy this simple and flavorful grilled asparagus with lemon and Parmesan as a tasty side dish! It's the perfect addition to any summer barbecue or weeknight dinner.

25. Chicken and vegetable stir-fry with brown rice

Ingredients:

- 1 cup broccoli florets
- 1 cup snap or snow peas
- 1 cup sliced mushrooms
- 2 green onions, sliced
- 3 tbsp low-sodium soy sauce
- 1 tsp sesame oil
- Salt and pepper to taste

- 1 cup brown rice
- 1 lb boneless, skinless chicken breasts, cut into 1-inch cubes
- 2 tbsp olive oil, divided
- 2 cloves garlic, minced
- 1 tbsp grated fresh ginger
- 1 red bell pepper, sliced

Instructions:

1. Cook the brown rice according to package instructions.

2. Season the chicken with salt and pepper. Heat 1 tbsp olive oil in a large skillet or wok over high heat. Add the chicken and stir-fry for 4-5 minutes until lightly browned but not fully cooked through. Remove chicken from skillet.

3. Add remaining 1 tbsp olive oil to the skillet along with the garlic and ginger. Stir-fry for 30 seconds until fragrant.

4. Add the bell pepper, broccoli, peas, mushrooms and green onions. Stir-fry for 4-5 minutes until veggies are crisp-tender.

5. Return the partially cooked chicken and any juices to the skillet. Add the soy sauce and sesame oil. Stir-fry for 2-3 more minutes until chicken is fully cooked through.

6. Remove from heat and adjust seasoning with salt and pepper if needed. Serve the chicken and veggie stir-fry over the cooked brown rice.

This stir-fry is packed with lean protein from the chicken, fiber and nutrients from the vegetables, and wholesome brown rice. The garlic, ginger and soy sauce provide amazing Asian-inspired flavors. Using a wok or large skillet ensures the ingredients cook quickly while retaining their vibrant crunch.

You can easily customize this stir-fry by using your favorite veggies. Carrots, bean sprouts, baby corn, water chestnuts or bok choy would all work nicely. For extra heat, add some chili garlic sauce or sriracha. This makes a complete, better-than-takeout meal at home!

26. Mediterranean chickpea salad

Ingredients:
- 2 cans (15 ounces each) chickpeas, drained and rinsed
- 1 cucumber, diced
- 1 bell pepper (red, yellow, or orange), diced
- 1 pint cherry tomatoes, halved
- 1/4 red onion, thinly sliced
- 1/2 cup Kalamata olives, pitted and halved
- 1/4 cup chopped fresh parsley
- 1/4 cup chopped fresh mint
- 1/3 cup crumbled feta cheese (optional)
- 1/4 cup extra virgin olive oil
- 2 tablespoons red wine vinegar
- 1 clove garlic, minced
- Salt and pepper to taste
- Lemon wedges for serving (optional)

Instructions:

1. In a large mixing bowl, combine chickpeas, diced cucumber, diced bell pepper, halved cherry tomatoes, thinly sliced red onion, halved Kalamata olives, chopped fresh parsley, and chopped fresh mint.

2. If using, add crumbled feta cheese to the bowl.

3. In a small bowl, whisk together extra virgin olive oil, red wine vinegar, minced garlic, salt, and pepper to make the dressing.

4. Pour the dressing over the chickpea salad and toss until well combined.

5. Let the salad marinate in the refrigerator for at least 30 minutes to allow the flavors to meld.

6. Before serving, taste and adjust the seasoning if needed.

7. Serve the Mediterranean chickpea salad chilled, garnished with lemon wedges if desired.

Enjoy this refreshing and flavorful Mediterranean chickpea salad as a light and healthy meal or side dish! It's packed with protein, fiber, and vibrant Mediterranean flavors.

27. Baked cod with tomatoes and olives

Ingredients:
- 4 cod fillets (about 6 ounces each)
- 2 tablespoons olive oil
- 2 cloves garlic, minced
- 1 pint cherry tomatoes, halved
- 1/2 cup Kalamata olives, pitted and halved
- 1 tablespoon capers, drained
- 1 teaspoon dried oregano
- Salt and pepper to taste
- Lemon wedges for serving
- Fresh parsley, chopped (for garnish)

Instructions:
1. Preheat your oven to 400°F (200°C). Lightly grease a baking dish with olive oil or cooking spray.

2. Place the cod fillets in the prepared baking dish.

3. In a small bowl, mix together olive oil, minced garlic, dried oregano, salt, and pepper.

4. Drizzle the olive oil mixture over the cod fillets, making sure to coat them evenly.

5. Scatter halved cherry tomatoes, halved Kalamata olives, and drained capers around the cod fillets in the baking dish.

6. Bake in the preheated oven for 12-15 minutes, or until the cod is opaque and flakes easily with a fork.

7. If desired, broil the cod for an additional 1-2 minutes at the end to brown the top slightly.

8. Remove the baked cod from the oven and let it rest for a few minutes.

9. Serve the baked cod hot, garnished with chopped fresh parsley and lemon wedges on the side for squeezing over the fish.

Enjoy this delicious and Mediterranean-inspired baked cod with tomatoes and olives! It's a simple yet flavorful dish that's perfect for a weeknight dinner.

28. Turkey and vegetable meatballs with zucchini noodles

Ingredients:
For the Meatballs:
- 1 lb ground turkey
- 1/2 cup breadcrumbs

For the Zucchini Noodles:
- 4 medium zucchini, spiralized
- 2 tablespoons olive oil
- 2 cloves garlic, minced
- Salt and pepper to taste

- 1/4 cup grated Parmesan cheese
- 1 egg
- 1/4 cup finely chopped onion
- 1/4 cup grated carrot
- 1/4 cup finely chopped bell pepper
- 2 cloves garlic, minced
- 1 teaspoon dried oregano
- 1 teaspoon dried basil
- Salt and pepper to taste
- Olive oil for cooking

Instructions:
For the Meatballs:
1. Preheat your oven to 375°F (190°C). Line a baking sheet with parchment paper.

2. In a large mixing bowl, combine ground turkey, breadcrumbs, grated Parmesan cheese, egg, chopped onion, grated carrot, chopped bell pepper, minced garlic, dried oregano, dried basil, salt, and pepper. Mix until well combined.

3. Shape the mixture into meatballs, about 1 inch in diameter, and place them on the prepared baking sheet.

4. Bake in the preheated oven for 20-25 minutes, or until the meatballs are cooked through and golden brown.

For the Zucchini Noodles:
1. While the meatballs are baking, heat olive oil in a large skillet over medium heat.

2. Add minced garlic to the skillet and cook for about 1 minute until fragrant.

3. Add spiralized zucchini noodles to the skillet. Cook for 2-3 minutes, tossing occasionally, until the noodles are just tender but still crisp. Season the zucchini noodles with salt and pepper to taste.

Serving:
1. Serve the turkey and vegetable meatballs over the zucchini noodles.

2. Optionally, garnish with grated Parmesan cheese and chopped fresh herbs like parsley or basil.

3. Enjoy your delicious and nutritious turkey and vegetable meatballs with zucchini noodles!

29. Grilled peach and arugula salad with balsamic dressing

Ingredients:
- 2 ripe peaches, halved and pitted
- 4 cups baby arugula
- 1/4 cup chopped walnuts or pecans
- 1/4 cup crumbled goat cheese or feta cheese
- Balsamic glaze (store-bought or homemade)
- Olive oil for grilling
- Salt and pepper to taste

For the Balsamic Dressing:
- 3 tablespoons balsamic vinegar
- 2 tablespoons extra virgin olive oil
- 1 teaspoon honey or maple syrup
- 1 teaspoon Dijon mustard
- Salt and pepper to taste

Instructions:

1. Preheat your grill to medium-high heat.

2. Brush the halved peaches with olive oil and sprinkle with a pinch of salt and pepper.

3. Place the peaches on the grill, cut side down, and grill for 3-4 minutes, or until grill marks appear and the peaches are slightly softened.

4. Remove the grilled peaches from the grill and let them cool slightly before slicing.

5. In a large mixing bowl, combine baby arugula, chopped walnuts or pecans, and crumbled goat cheese or feta cheese.

6. Arrange the grilled peach slices on top of the arugula mixture.

7. In a small bowl, whisk together balsamic vinegar, extra virgin olive oil, honey or maple syrup, Dijon mustard, salt, and pepper to make the dressing.

8. Drizzle the balsamic dressing over the salad.

9. Optionally, drizzle balsamic glaze over the salad for extra sweetness and flavor.

10. Toss the salad gently to coat everything evenly.

11. Serve immediately and enjoy your delicious grilled peach and arugula salad!

This salad is a perfect combination of sweet, savory, and tangy flavors, with the added crunch of nuts. It's a refreshing and elegant dish that's perfect for summer gatherings or as a light lunch or dinner option.

30. Vegetarian stuffed peppers with quinoa and black beans

Ingredients:
- 4 large bell peppers, any color
- 1 cup quinoa, rinsed
- 1 can (15 ounces) black beans, drained and rinsed
- 1 cup corn kernels (fresh, frozen, or canned)
- 1/2 onion, finely chopped
- 2 cloves garlic, minced
- 1 teaspoon ground cumin
- 1 teaspoon chili powder
- 1/2 teaspoon smoked paprika
- Salt and pepper to taste
- 1 cup shredded cheese (cheddar, Monterey Jack, or Mexican blend)
- Fresh cilantro, chopped (for garnish)
- Lime wedges (for serving)

Instructions:
1. Preheat your oven to 375°F (190°C).
Grease a baking dish large enough to hold the stuffed peppers.

2. Cut the tops off the bell peppers and remove the seeds and membranes. Place the peppers upright in the prepared baking dish.

3. In a medium saucepan, bring 2 cups of water to a boil. Add the rinsed quinoa, reduce the heat to low, cover, and simmer for about 15 minutes, or until the quinoa is cooked and the water is absorbed. Remove from heat and fluff with a fork.

4. In a large skillet, heat some olive oil over medium heat. Add chopped onion and cook until softened, about 3-4 minutes. Add minced garlic and cook for another minute.

5. Add cooked quinoa, black beans, corn kernels, ground cumin, chili powder, smoked paprika, salt, and pepper to the skillet. Stir well to combine and cook for a few more minutes until heated through.

6. Remove the skillet from heat and stir in half of the shredded cheese.

7. Spoon the quinoa and black bean mixture into the hollowed-out bell peppers, pressing down gently to pack the filling.

8. Cover the baking dish with aluminum foil and bake in the preheated oven for 25-30 minutes, or until the peppers are tender.

9. Remove the foil, sprinkle the remaining shredded cheese over the stuffed peppers, and return them to the oven for another 5 minutes, or until the cheese is melted and bubbly.

10. Remove from the oven and let the stuffed peppers cool for a few minutes before serving. Garnish with chopped fresh cilantro and serve with lime wedges on the side.

31. Baked salmon with pineapple salsa

Ingredients:
- 4 salmon fillets (about 6 ounces each)
- Salt and pepper to taste
- 1 tablespoon olive oil
- 1 teaspoon paprika
- 1 teaspoon garlic powder
- 1 cup diced pineapple
- 1/4 cup diced red bell pepper
- 1/4 cup diced red onion
- 1 jalapeño pepper, seeded and minced
- Juice of 1 lime
- 2 tablespoons chopped fresh cilantro
- Salt to taste

Instructions:
1. Preheat your oven to 375°F (190°C).

2. Season the salmon fillets with salt and pepper to taste.

3. In a small bowl, mix together the olive oil, paprika, and garlic powder.

4. Brush the olive oil mixture over the salmon fillets.

5. Place the seasoned salmon fillets on a baking sheet lined with parchment paper.

6. Bake in the preheated oven for 12-15 minutes, or until the salmon is cooked through and flakes easily with a fork.

7. While the salmon is baking, prepare the pineapple salsa. In a medium bowl, combine the diced pineapple, diced red bell pepper, diced red onion, minced jalapeño pepper, lime juice, chopped cilantro, and salt to taste. Mix well.

8. Once the salmon is done baking, remove it from the oven and let it cool slightly. Serve the baked salmon topped with the pineapple salsa.

9. Garnish with additional cilantro if desired. Enjoy your delicious Baked Salmon with Pineapple Salsa!

This dish is bursting with flavor and makes for a perfect combination of sweet and savory. It's sure to be a hit at any dinner table!

32. Tuna and white bean salad

Ingredients:
- 2 cans (5 ounces each) of tuna, drained
- 2 cans (15 ounces each) of white beans (such as cannellini or navy beans), drained and rinsed
- 1/4 cup red onion, finely chopped
- 1/4 cup fresh parsley, chopped
- 1/4 cup celery, finely chopped
- 1/4 cup red bell pepper, finely chopped
- 2 tablespoons capers, drained
- 2 tablespoons lemon juice
- 2 tablespoons extra virgin olive oil
- Salt and pepper to taste
- Optional: cherry tomatoes, cucumber slices, mixed salad greens for serving

Instructions:
1. In a large mixing bowl, combine the drained tuna, white beans, chopped red onion, chopped parsley, chopped celery, chopped red bell pepper, and capers.

2. In a small bowl, whisk together the lemon juice and extra virgin olive oil to make the dressing.

3. Pour the dressing over the tuna and white bean mixture in the large bowl.

4. Gently toss everything together until well combined.

5. Season the salad with salt and pepper to taste, adjusting as needed.

6. Optional: Serve the tuna and white bean salad over a bed of mixed salad greens and garnish with cherry tomatoes and cucumber slices.

7. Enjoy your delicious and protein-packed Tuna and White Bean Salad!

This salad is not only healthy and nutritious but also flavorful and satisfying. It's perfect for a light lunch or dinner, and it can also be prepared ahead of time for meal prep.

33. Grilled chicken with mango and avocado salsa

Ingredients:
For the Grilled Chicken:
- 4 boneless, skinless chicken breasts
- 2 tablespoons olive oil
- Salt and pepper to taste
- 1 teaspoon paprika
- 1 teaspoon garlic powder
- 1 teaspoon onion powder

For the Mango and Avocado Salsa:
- 1 ripe mango, diced
- 1 ripe avocado, diced
- 1/4 cup red onion, finely chopped
- 1 jalapeño pepper, seeded and minced
- Juice of 1 lime
- 2 tablespoons chopped fresh cilantro
- Salt and pepper to taste

Instructions:
For the Grilled Chicken:
1. Preheat your grill to medium-high heat.

2. In a small bowl, mix together olive oil, salt, pepper, paprika, garlic powder, and onion powder to create a marinade.

3. Brush the chicken breasts with the marinade, coating them evenly.

4. Grill the chicken breasts for about 6-8 minutes per side, or until they are cooked through and have nice grill marks. Cooking time may vary depending on the thickness of the chicken breasts.

5. Once cooked, remove the chicken breasts from the grill and let them rest for a few minutes before serving.

For the Mango and Avocado Salsa:
1. In a medium bowl, combine diced mango, diced avocado, finely chopped red onion, minced jalapeño pepper, lime juice, chopped cilantro, salt, and pepper. Mix well. Taste and adjust the seasoning, if needed.

Serving:
1. Place grilled chicken breasts on plates or a platter. Spoon the mango and avocado salsa over the grilled chicken breasts.

3. Garnish with additional cilantro, if desired. Serve immediately and enjoy your Grilled Chicken with Mango and Avocado Salsa!

This dish is bursting with fresh flavors and vibrant colors, making it perfect for a summer barbecue or weeknight dinner. The combination of juicy grilled chicken and sweet-spicy mango and avocado salsa is sure to impress!

34. Roasted cauliflower and chickpea salad

Ingredients:
- 1 head cauliflower, cut into florets
- 1 can (15 ounces) chickpeas, drained and rinsed
- 2 tablespoons olive oil
- 1 teaspoon ground cumin
- 1 teaspoon smoked paprika
- 1/2 teaspoon garlic powder
- Salt and pepper to taste
- 4 cups mixed salad greens
- 1/4 cup chopped fresh parsley
- 1/4 cup crumbled feta cheese (optional)

For the Dressing:
- 3 tablespoons olive oil
- 2 tablespoons lemon juice
- 1 teaspoon Dijon mustard
- 1 clove garlic, minced
- Salt and pepper to taste

Instructions:

1. Preheat your oven to 400°F (200°C). Line a baking sheet with parchment paper.

2. In a large bowl, toss the cauliflower florets and chickpeas with olive oil, ground cumin, smoked paprika, garlic powder, salt, and pepper until evenly coated.

3. Spread the seasoned cauliflower and chickpeas in a single layer on the prepared baking sheet.

4. Roast in the preheated oven for 25-30 minutes, stirring halfway through, until the cauliflower is tender and lightly browned.

5. While the cauliflower and chickpeas are roasting, prepare the dressing. In a small bowl, whisk together olive oil, lemon juice, Dijon mustard, minced garlic, salt, and pepper until well combined.

6. Once the cauliflower and chickpeas are done roasting, remove them from the oven and let them cool slightly.

7. In a large mixing bowl, combine the roasted cauliflower and chickpeas with mixed salad greens and chopped fresh parsley.

8. Drizzle the dressing over the salad and toss until everything is well coated.

9. If using, sprinkle crumbled feta cheese over the salad.

10. Serve the roasted cauliflower and chickpea salad immediately, either as a side dish or a light meal.

35. Lentil and vegetable soup

Ingredients:
- 1 cup dried green or
brown lentils, rinsed and drained
- 1 onion, chopped
- 2 carrots, chopped
- 2 celery stalks, chopped
- 2 cloves garlic, minced
- 1 can (14.5 ounces) diced tomatoes
- 4 cups vegetable broth
- 2 cups water
- 1 teaspoon dried thyme
- 1 teaspoon dried oregano
- 1 bay leaf
- Salt and pepper to taste
- 2 cups chopped fresh spinach or kale
- 2 tablespoons chopped fresh parsley (for garnish)
- Lemon wedges (optional, for serving)

Instructions:

1. In a large pot or Dutch oven, heat a bit of olive oil over medium heat.

2. Add chopped onion, carrots, and celery to the pot. Cook, stirring occasionally, for about 5 minutes until the vegetables start to soften.

3. Add minced garlic to the pot and cook for an additional minute until fragrant.

4. Stir in the rinsed lentils, diced tomatoes (with their juices), vegetable broth, water, dried thyme, dried oregano, bay leaf, salt, and pepper.

5. Bring the soup to a boil, then reduce the heat to low. Cover and simmer for about 20-25 minutes, or until the lentils are tender.

6. Once the lentils are cooked, stir in the chopped fresh spinach or kale. Cook for a few more minutes until the greens are wilted.

7. Taste and adjust the seasoning with more salt and pepper if needed. Remove the bay leaf from the soup before serving.

9. Ladle the lentil and vegetable soup into bowls. Garnish with chopped fresh parsley. Optionally, serve the soup with lemon wedges on the side for squeezing over each bowl before eating.

Enjoy this comforting and nutritious Lentil and Vegetable Soup! It's perfect for a cozy meal on a chilly day and makes excellent leftovers for lunch the next day.

36. Grilled shrimp and vegetable skewers

Ingredients:
- 1 lb large shrimp, peeled and deveined
- 2 zucchinis, sliced into rounds
- 1 red bell pepper, cut into chunks
- 1 yellow bell pepper, cut into chunks
- 1 red onion, cut into chunks
- 8-10 cherry tomatoes
- 8-10 wooden skewers, soaked in water for 30 minutes
- Olive oil, for brushing
- Salt and pepper to taste
- Lemon wedges (for serving)
- Fresh parsley, chopped (for garnish)

For the Marinade:
- 1/4 cup olive oil
- 2 cloves garlic, minced
- 1 teaspoon lemon zest
- 2 tablespoons lemon juice
- 1 teaspoon dried oregano
- 1 teaspoon dried basil
- Salt and pepper to taste

Instructions:

1. In a small bowl, whisk together all the ingredients for the marinade.

2. Place the shrimp in a shallow dish and pour half of the marinade over them. Toss to coat evenly. Cover and refrigerate for 20-30 minutes.

3. Preheat your grill to medium-high heat.

4. Thread the marinated shrimp, zucchini slices, bell pepper chunks, onion chunks, and cherry tomatoes onto the soaked skewers, alternating between ingredients.

5. Brush the assembled skewers with olive oil and season with salt and pepper.

6. Place the skewers on the preheated grill and cook for 2-3 minutes per side, or until the shrimp are pink and opaque and the vegetables are charred and tender.

7. Once cooked, remove the skewers from the grill and transfer them to a serving platter.

8. Drizzle the remaining marinade over the skewers and garnish with chopped fresh parsley.

9. Serve the grilled shrimp and vegetable skewers hot, with lemon wedges on the side for squeezing over the top.

37. Turkey and vegetable chili

Ingredients:
- 1 lb ground turkey
- 1 tablespoon olive oil
- 1 onion, chopped
- 2 cloves garlic, minced
- 1 bell pepper, diced
- 1 zucchini, diced
- 1 carrot, diced
- 1 can (14.5 ounces) diced tomatoes
- 1 can (15 ounces) kidney beans, drained and rinsed
- 1 can (15 ounces) black beans, drained and rinsed
- 2 cups vegetable broth
- 2 tablespoons tomato paste
- 1 tablespoon chili powder
- 1 teaspoon ground cumin
- 1 teaspoon dried oregano
- Salt and pepper to taste
- Optional toppings: shredded cheese, sour cream, chopped green onions, cilantro

Instructions:

1. Heat olive oil in a large pot or Dutch oven over medium heat.

2. Add chopped onion and minced garlic to the pot. Cook until softened and fragrant, about 2-3 minutes.

3. Add ground turkey to the pot. Cook, breaking it apart with a spoon, until browned and cooked through.

4. Stir in diced bell pepper, diced zucchini, and diced carrot. Cook for another 5-7 minutes, until the vegetables start to soften.

5. Add diced tomatoes (with their juices), drained and rinsed kidney beans, drained and rinsed black beans, vegetable broth, tomato paste, chili powder, ground cumin, dried oregano, salt, and pepper to the pot. Stir well to combine.

6. Bring the chili to a simmer, then reduce the heat to low. Cover and let it simmer for about 20-25 minutes, stirring occasionally.

7. Taste and adjust the seasoning with more salt and pepper if needed.

8. Serve the turkey and vegetable chili hot, topped with your favorite toppings such as shredded cheese, sour cream, chopped green onions, or cilantro.

Enjoy this flavorful and nutritious Turkey and Vegetable Chili! It's perfect for warming up on a chilly day and makes excellent leftovers for meal prep.

38. Spinach and feta stuffed mushrooms

Ingredients:
- 16 large white or cremini mushrooms, stems removed
- 1 tablespoon olive oil
- 1 small onion, finely chopped
- 2 cloves garlic, minced
- 4 cups fresh spinach leaves, chopped
- 1/4 cup breadcrumbs
- 1/2 cup crumbled feta cheese
- 1/4 cup grated Parmesan cheese
- 1 tablespoon fresh parsley, chopped
- Salt and pepper to taste
- Cooking spray or additional olive oil for greasing the baking sheet

Instructions:
1. Preheat your oven to 375°F (190°C). Lightly grease a baking sheet with cooking spray or olive oil.

2. Clean the mushrooms and remove the stems. Set the mushroom caps aside.

3. Finely chop the mushroom stems.

4. In a large skillet, heat the olive oil over medium heat. Add the chopped onion and cook until softened, about 3-4 minutes.

5. Add the minced garlic and cook for another minute until fragrant.

6. Stir in the chopped mushroom stems and cook for about 2-3 minutes until they start to release their moisture.

7. Add the chopped spinach and cook until wilted, about 2-3 minutes.

8. Remove the skillet from heat and stir in the breadcrumbs, crumbled feta cheese, grated Parmesan cheese, chopped parsley, salt, and pepper. Mix until well combined.

9. Spoon the spinach and feta mixture into the mushroom caps, pressing gently to pack the filling. Place the stuffed mushrooms on the prepared baking sheet.

10. Bake in the preheated oven for 20-25 minutes, or until the mushrooms are tender and the tops are golden brown. Remove from the oven and let cool slightly before serving.

39. Baked cod with tomatoes and basil

Ingredients:
- 4 cod fillets (about 6 ounces each)
- 2 tablespoons olive oil
- 1 pint cherry tomatoes, halved
- 3 cloves garlic, minced
- 1/4 cup fresh basil leaves, chopped
- 1 lemon, thinly sliced
- Salt and pepper to taste
- Lemon wedges (for serving)

Instructions:

1. Preheat your oven to 375°F (190°C). Lightly grease a baking dish with olive oil.

2. Place the cod fillets in the prepared baking dish. Season them with salt and pepper to taste.

3. In a medium bowl, combine the halved cherry tomatoes, minced garlic, chopped basil, and 1 tablespoon of olive oil. Mix well.

4. Spoon the tomato mixture evenly over and around the cod fillets.

5. Arrange the thin lemon slices on top of and around the fish.

6. Drizzle the remaining 1 tablespoon of olive oil over the entire dish.

7. Bake in the preheated oven for 20-25 minutes, or until the cod is opaque and flakes easily with a fork.

8. Remove from the oven and let the dish cool slightly.

9. Serve the baked cod with additional lemon wedges on the side.

Enjoy this light and healthy Baked Cod with Tomatoes and Basil! It's a perfect weeknight dinner that's both easy to prepare and full of fresh flavors.

40. Quinoa and roasted vegetable bowls

Ingredients:
- 1 cup quinoa, rinsed
- 2 cups water or vegetable broth

For the Dressing:
- 3 tablespoons olive oil
- 2 tablespoons lemon juice
- 1 teaspoon Dijon mustard
- 1 clove garlic, minced
- Salt and pepper to taste

- 1 red bell pepper, diced
- 1 yellow bell pepper, diced
- 1 zucchini, diced
- 1 red onion, diced
- 1 cup cherry tomatoes, halved
- 1 cup broccoli florets
- 3 tablespoons olive oil, divided
- Salt and pepper to taste
- 1 teaspoon dried oregano
- 1 teaspoon garlic powder
- 1/4 cup fresh parsley, chopped (for garnish)
- Optional toppings: crumbled feta cheese, avocado slices, hummus

Instructions:
1. Preheat your oven to 400°F (200°C). Line a baking sheet with parchment paper.

2. In a medium saucepan, bring 2 cups of water or vegetable broth to a boil. Add the rinsed quinoa, reduce the heat to low, cover, and simmer for about 15 minutes, or until the quinoa is cooked and the water is absorbed. Remove from heat and fluff with a fork.

3. In a large bowl, combine the diced red bell pepper, yellow bell pepper, zucchini, red onion, cherry tomatoes, and broccoli florets. Drizzle with 2 tablespoons of olive oil, and season with salt, pepper, dried oregano, and garlic powder. Toss to coat evenly.

4. Spread the seasoned vegetables in a single layer on the prepared baking sheet. Roast in the preheated oven for 20-25 minutes, or until the vegetables are tender and slightly browned.

5. While the vegetables are roasting, prepare the dressing. In a small bowl, whisk together 3 tablespoons of olive oil, lemon juice, Dijon mustard, minced garlic, salt, and pepper until well combined.

6. Once the vegetables are done roasting, remove them from the oven and let them cool slightly.

7. To assemble the bowls, divide the cooked quinoa among four bowls. Top each bowl with a portion of the roasted vegetables.

8. Drizzle the dressing over each bowl and garnish with chopped fresh parsley. Add optional toppings like crumbled feta cheese, avocado slices, or a dollop of hummus if desired.

41. Grilled salmon with mango salsa

Ingredients:

For the Grilled Salmon:
- 4 salmon fillets (about 6 ounces each)
- 2 tablespoons olive oil
- Salt and pepper to taste
- 1 teaspoon paprika
- 1 teaspoon garlic powder

For the Mango Salsa:
- 1 ripe mango, diced
- 1/4 cup red bell pepper, diced
- 1/4 cup red onion, finely chopped
- 1 jalapeño pepper, seeded and minced
- Juice of 1 lime
- 2 tablespoons fresh cilantro, chopped
- Salt to taste

Instructions:

For the Grilled Salmon:

1. Preheat your grill to medium-high heat.

2. In a small bowl, mix together the olive oil, salt, pepper, paprika, and garlic powder.

3. Brush the salmon fillets with the olive oil mixture, coating them evenly.

4. Place the salmon fillets on the preheated grill. Grill for about 4-6 minutes per side, or until the salmon is cooked through and has nice grill marks. The salmon should be opaque and flake easily with a fork.

For the Mango Salsa:

1. In a medium bowl, combine the diced mango, red bell pepper, red onion, minced jalapeño pepper, lime juice, chopped cilantro, and salt. Mix well.

2. Taste and adjust the seasoning if needed.

To Serve:

1. Place the grilled salmon fillets on plates.

2. Spoon the mango salsa over the salmon fillets.

3. Garnish with additional cilantro if desired.

4. Serve immediately.

42. Turkey and vegetable lettuce wraps

Ingredients:
- 1 lb ground turkey
- 1 tablespoon olive oil
- 1 small onion, finely chopped
- 2 cloves garlic, minced
- 1 red bell pepper, diced
- 1 carrot, grated
- 1 zucchini, diced
- 1/4 cup hoisin sauce
- 2 tablespoons soy sauce
(or tamari for gluten-free)
- 1 tablespoon rice vinegar
- 1 teaspoon grated fresh ginger
- Salt and pepper to taste
- 1 head butter lettuce or iceberg lettuce, leaves separated
- Optional toppings: chopped green onions, sesame seeds, chopped fresh cilantro, sriracha

Instructions:

1. In a large skillet, heat the olive oil over medium heat.

2. Add the finely chopped onion and cook until softened, about 3-4 minutes.

3. Add the minced garlic and cook for another minute until fragrant.

4. Add the ground turkey to the skillet. Cook, breaking it up with a spoon, until browned and cooked through.

5. Stir in the diced red bell pepper, grated carrot, and diced zucchini. Cook for about 5 minutes until the vegetables are tender.

6. In a small bowl, whisk together the hoisin sauce, soy sauce, rice vinegar, and grated fresh ginger.

7. Pour the sauce over the turkey and vegetable mixture in the skillet. Stir well to combine and cook for another 2-3 minutes, allowing the flavors to meld. Season with salt and pepper to taste.

8. Remove from heat and let the mixture cool slightly.

9. To serve, spoon the turkey and vegetable mixture into the center of each lettuce leaf.

10. Top with optional toppings such as chopped green onions, sesame seeds, chopped fresh cilantro, and a drizzle of sriracha for extra heat.

43. Lentil and sweet potato stew

Ingredients:
- 1 cup dried green or brown lentils, rinsed and drained
- 2 tablespoons olive oil
- 1 onion, chopped
- 2 cloves garlic, minced
- 2 medium sweet potatoes, peeled and diced
- 2 carrots, sliced
- 2 celery stalks, sliced
- 1 red bell pepper, diced
- 1 can (14.5 ounces) diced tomatoes
- 4 cups vegetable broth
- 1 teaspoon ground cumin
- 1 teaspoon ground coriander
- 1 teaspoon smoked paprika
- 1/2 teaspoon ground cinnamon
- Salt and pepper to taste
- 2 cups chopped kale or spinach
- 1/4 cup chopped fresh parsley (for garnish)

Instructions:
1. In a large pot or Dutch oven, heat the olive oil over medium heat.

2. Add the chopped onion and cook until softened, about 5 minutes.

3. Add the minced garlic and cook for another minute until fragrant.

4. Stir in the diced sweet potatoes, sliced carrots, sliced celery, and diced red bell pepper. Cook for about 5 minutes, stirring occasionally.

5. Add the lentils, diced tomatoes (with their juices), vegetable broth, ground cumin, ground coriander, smoked paprika, ground cinnamon, salt, and pepper. Stir well to combine.

6. Bring the stew to a boil, then reduce the heat to low. Cover and simmer for about 30 minutes, or until the lentils and vegetables are tender.

7. Stir in the chopped kale or spinach and cook for an additional 5 minutes, until the greens are wilted.

8. Taste and adjust the seasoning with more salt and pepper if needed. Serve the lentil and sweet potato stew hot, garnished with chopped fresh parsley

44. Roasted Brussels sprouts with balsamic glaze

Ingredients:
- 1 lb Brussels sprouts, trimmed and halved
- 2 tablespoons olive oil
- Salt and pepper to taste
- 1/4 cup balsamic vinegar
- 1 tablespoon honey or maple syrup

Instructions:
1. Preheat your oven to 400°F (200°C). Line a baking sheet with parchment paper or lightly grease it.

2. In a large bowl, toss the halved Brussels sprouts with olive oil, salt, and pepper until evenly coated.

3. Spread the Brussels sprouts in a single layer on the prepared baking sheet, cut side down.
4. Roast in the preheated oven for 20-25 minutes, or until the Brussels sprouts are tender and caramelized, stirring halfway through for even roasting.

5. While the Brussels sprouts are roasting, prepare the balsamic glaze. In a small saucepan, combine the balsamic vinegar and honey (or maple syrup).

6. Bring the mixture to a simmer over medium heat, then reduce the heat to low and simmer for about 5-7 minutes, or until the mixture has thickened to a syrupy consistency. Remove from heat and let cool slightly.

7. Once the Brussels sprouts are done roasting, transfer them to a serving dish.

8. Drizzle the balsamic glaze over the roasted Brussels sprouts and toss to coat evenly.

9. Serve immediately.

Enjoy these flavorful Roasted Brussels Sprouts with Balsamic Glaze as a delicious side dish! They are perfect for adding a touch of elegance and a burst of flavor to any meal.

45. Baked tilapia with tomatoes and olives

Ingredients:
- 4 tilapia fillets (about 6 ounces each)
- 2 tablespoons olive oil
- 1 pint cherry tomatoes, halved
- 1/2 cup Kalamata olives, pitted and halved
- 1 small red onion, thinly sliced
- 3 cloves garlic, minced
- 1 lemon, thinly sliced
- 1 teaspoon dried oregano
- Salt and pepper to taste
- Fresh parsley, chopped (for garnish)
- Lemon wedges (for serving)

Instructions:
1. Preheat your oven to 375°F (190°C). Lightly grease a baking dish with olive oil.

2. Place the tilapia fillets in the baking dish. Season them with salt, pepper, and dried oregano.

3. In a medium bowl, combine the halved cherry tomatoes, Kalamata olives, thinly sliced red onion, and minced garlic. Mix well.

4. Spoon the tomato and olive mixture evenly over and around the tilapia fillets.

5. Arrange the lemon slices on top of and around the fish.

6. Drizzle 2 tablespoons of olive oil over the entire dish.

7. Bake in the preheated oven for 20-25 minutes, or until the tilapia is opaque and flakes easily with a fork.

8. Remove from the oven and let the dish cool slightly.

9. Garnish with chopped fresh parsley.

10. Serve the baked tilapia with additional lemon wedges on the side.

Enjoy this flavorful and Mediterranean-inspired Baked Tilapia with Tomatoes and Olives! It's perfect for a healthy and quick weeknight dinner.

46. Greek salad with grilled chicken

Ingredients:
For the Grilled Chicken:
- 2 boneless, skinless chicken breasts
- 2 tablespoons olive oil
- 1 teaspoon dried oregano
- 1 teaspoon garlic powder
- Salt and pepper to taste
- Juice of 1 lemon

For the Greek Salad:
- 6 cups romaine lettuce, chopped
- 1 cucumber, sliced
- 1 pint cherry tomatoes, halved
- 1 red bell pepper, diced
- 1/2 red onion, thinly sliced
- 1/2 cup Kalamata olives, pitted
- 1/2 cup feta cheese, crumbled

Instructions:
For the Grilled Chicken:
1. In a small bowl, mix together the olive oil, dried oregano, garlic powder, salt, pepper, and lemon juice.

2. Place the chicken breasts in a resealable plastic bag or shallow dish and pour the marinade over them. Marinate for at least 30 minutes, or up to 2 hours.

3. Preheat your grill to medium-high heat.

4. Grill the chicken breasts for 6-7 minutes per side, or until fully cooked and the internal temperature reaches 165°F (74°C). Remove from the grill and let rest for a few minutes before slicing.

For the Dressing:
- 1/4 cup olive oil
- 2 tablespoons red wine vinegar
- 1 teaspoon dried oregano
- 1 teaspoon Dijon mustard
- 1 clove garlic, minced
- Salt and pepper to taste

For the Greek Salad: In a large bowl, combine the chopped romaine lettuce, sliced cucumber, halved cherry tomatoes, diced red bell pepper, thinly sliced red onion, Kalamata olives, and crumbled feta cheese.

For the Dressing: In a small bowl, whisk together the olive oil, red wine vinegar, dried oregano, Dijon mustard, minced garlic, salt, and pepper until well combined.

To Assemble: Drizzle the dressing over the salad and toss to coat evenly. Top the salad with the sliced grilled chicken. Serve immediately.

47. Turkey and vegetable meatballs with zucchini noodles

Ingredients:
For the Turkey and Vegetable Meatballs:
- 1 lb ground turkey
- Salt and pepper to taste
- Olive oil for cooking

For the Zucchini Noodles:
- 4 medium zucchini, spiralized into noodles
- 2 tablespoons olive oil
- 2 cloves garlic, minced
- Salt and pepper to taste

- 1/2 cup grated zucchini, squeezed to remove excess moisture
- 1/4 cup grated carrot
- 1/4 cup finely chopped onion
- 2 cloves garlic, minced
- 1/4 cup breadcrumbs (or almond flour for a gluten-free option)
- 1 egg
- 2 tablespoons chopped fresh parsley
- 1 teaspoon dried oregano
- 1/2 teaspoon paprika

Instructions:
For the Turkey and Vegetable Meatballs:
1. Preheat your oven to 400°F (200°C). Line a baking sheet with parchment paper.

2. In a large mixing bowl, combine the ground turkey, grated zucchini, grated carrot, chopped onion, minced garlic, breadcrumbs, egg, chopped parsley, dried oregano, paprika, salt, and pepper. Mix until well combined.

3. Shape the mixture into meatballs, about 1-2 tablespoons each, and place them on the prepared baking sheet.

4. Bake in the preheated oven for 20-25 minutes, or until the meatballs are cooked through and lightly browned.

For the Zucchini Noodles:
1. While the meatballs are baking, heat olive oil in a large skillet over medium heat.
2. Add minced garlic to the skillet and cook for about 1 minute until fragrant.
3. Add the spiralized zucchini noodles to the skillet and toss to coat in the garlic-infused oil. Cook for 2-3 minutes until the noodles are just tender but still crisp.
4. Season the zucchini noodles with salt and pepper to taste.

To Serve:
1. Divide the zucchini noodles among serving plates or bowls.
2. Top the zucchini noodles with the cooked turkey and vegetable meatballs.
3. Optionally, garnish with additional chopped parsley or grated Parmesan cheese.
4. Serve immediately and enjoy!

48. Roasted cauliflower and chickpea tacos

Ingredients:
For the Roasted Cauliflower and Chickpeas:
- 1 head cauliflower, cut into florets
- 1 can (15 ounces) chickpeas, drained and rinsed
- 2 tablespoons olive oil
- 1 teaspoon ground cumin
- 1 teaspoon smoked paprika
- 1/2 teaspoon garlic powder
- Salt and pepper to taste

For the Tacos:
- 8 small corn or flour tortillas
- 1 avocado, sliced
- 1/4 cup chopped fresh cilantro
- 1 lime, cut into wedges
- Hot sauce or salsa (optional, for serving)

Instructions:
For the Roasted Cauliflower and Chickpeas:
1. Preheat your oven to 400°F (200°C). Line a baking sheet with parchment paper.

2. In a large bowl, toss the cauliflower florets and chickpeas with olive oil, ground cumin, smoked paprika, garlic powder, salt, and pepper until evenly coated.

3. Spread the seasoned cauliflower and chickpeas in a single layer on the prepared baking sheet.

4. Roast in the preheated oven for 25-30 minutes, or until the cauliflower is tender and lightly browned, and the chickpeas are crispy, stirring halfway through for even cooking.

For the Tacos:
1. Warm the tortillas in a dry skillet or microwave according to package instructions.

2. Divide the roasted cauliflower and chickpeas among the warm tortillas.

3. Top each taco with sliced avocado and chopped fresh cilantro.

4. Serve with lime wedges and hot sauce or salsa on the side, if desired.

Enjoy these flavorful and satisfying Roasted Cauliflower and Chickpea Tacos! They're perfect for a meatless dinner option that's packed with protein and fiber.

49. Grilled peach and arugula salad with balsamic dressing

Ingredients:
- 4 ripe peaches, halved and pitted
- 6 cups arugula
- 1/2 cup crumbled feta cheese
- 1/4 cup chopped pecans or walnuts
- 2 tablespoons extra virgin olive oil
- 2 tablespoons balsamic vinegar
- 1 teaspoon honey or maple syrup
- Salt and pepper to taste

Instructions:

For Grilling the Peaches:
1. Preheat your grill to medium-high heat.

2. Brush the peach halves with a bit of olive oil to prevent sticking.

3. Place the peach halves on the grill, cut side down, and grill for 2-3 minutes until grill marks form. Flip and grill for an additional 2-3 minutes on the other side. Remove from the grill and let cool slightly.

For Assembling the Salad:
1. In a large bowl, combine the arugula, crumbled feta cheese, and chopped pecans or walnuts.

2. Slice the grilled peach halves into wedges and add them to the salad.

3. In a small bowl, whisk together the extra virgin olive oil, balsamic vinegar, honey or maple syrup, salt, and pepper to make the dressing.

4. Drizzle the dressing over the salad and toss gently to coat everything evenly.

Enjoy this flavorful and refreshing Grilled Peach and Arugula Salad with Balsamic Dressing! It's perfect for a light summer lunch or as a side dish for grilled meats.

50. Vegetarian chili with sweet potatoes and black beans

Ingredients:
- 2 tablespoons olive oil
- 1 large onion, diced
- 3 cloves garlic, minced
- 2 medium sweet potatoes, peeled and diced
- 1 red bell pepper, diced
- 1 yellow bell pepper, diced
- 2 carrots, diced
- 1 can (15 ounces) black beans, drained and rinsed
- 1 can (15 ounces) diced tomatoes
- 1 can (15 ounces) tomato sauce
- 2 cups vegetable broth
- 1 tablespoon chili powder
- 1 teaspoon ground cumin
- 1 teaspoon smoked paprika
- 1/2 teaspoon dried oregano
- Salt and pepper to taste
- Optional toppings: chopped fresh cilantro, sliced green onions, shredded cheese, sour cream, avocado slices

Instructions:
1. Heat the olive oil in a large pot or Dutch oven over medium heat.

2. Add the diced onion and cook until softened, about 5 minutes.

3. Add the minced garlic and cook for another minute until fragrant.

4. Add the diced sweet potatoes, diced bell peppers, and diced carrots to the pot. Cook for about 5 minutes, stirring occasionally.

5. Stir in the drained and rinsed black beans, diced tomatoes, tomato sauce, vegetable broth, chili powder, ground cumin, smoked paprika, dried oregano, salt, and pepper.

6. Bring the chili to a simmer, then reduce the heat to low. Cover and let it simmer for about 20-25 minutes, or until the sweet potatoes are tender, stirring occasionally.

7. Taste and adjust the seasoning with more salt and pepper if needed.

8. Serve the vegetarian chili hot, garnished with optional toppings such as chopped fresh cilantro, sliced green onions, shredded cheese, sour cream, or avocado slices.

51. Baked salmon with pineapple salsa

Ingredients:
For the Baked Salmon:
- 4 salmon fillets (about 6 ounces each)
- 2 tablespoons olive oil
- Salt and pepper to taste
- 1 teaspoon paprika
- 1 teaspoon garlic powder

For the Pineapple Salsa:
- 2 cups fresh pineapple, diced
- 1/4 cup red onion, finely chopped
- 1 jalapeño pepper, seeded and minced
- 1/4 cup chopped fresh cilantro
- Juice of 1 lime
- Salt and pepper to taste

Instructions:
For the Baked Salmon:
1. Preheat your oven to 375°F (190°C). Line a baking sheet with parchment paper.

2. Place the salmon fillets on the prepared baking sheet.

3. Drizzle the olive oil over the salmon fillets.

4. Season the salmon fillets with salt, pepper, paprika, and garlic powder.

5. Bake in the preheated oven for 12-15 minutes, or until the salmon is cooked through and flakes easily with a fork.

For the Pineapple Salsa:
1. In a medium bowl, combine the diced pineapple, finely chopped red onion, minced jalapeño pepper, chopped fresh cilantro, and lime juice.

2. Season the salsa with salt and pepper to taste. Mix well.

To Serve:
1. Once the salmon is done baking, transfer it to serving plates.

2. Spoon the pineapple salsa over the baked salmon fillets.

3. Serve immediately.

52. Tuna and white bean salad

Ingredients:
- 2 cans (5 ounces each) of tuna, drained
- 2 cans (15 ounces each) of cannellini beans, drained and rinsed
- 1/2 red onion, finely chopped
- 1/4 cup chopped fresh parsley
- 1/4 cup chopped fresh basil
- 2 tablespoons capers, drained
- 2 tablespoons extra virgin olive oil
- Juice of 1 lemon
- Salt and pepper to taste
- Optional: cherry tomatoes, sliced cucumber, olives

Instructions:
1. In a large mixing bowl, combine the drained tuna, cannellini beans, finely chopped red onion, chopped fresh parsley, chopped fresh basil, and capers.

2. Drizzle the extra virgin olive oil and lemon juice over the salad.

3. Season with salt and pepper to taste.

4. Gently toss the salad until all the ingredients are well combined.

5. Taste and adjust the seasoning if needed.

6. If desired, add cherry tomatoes, sliced cucumber, or olives for extra flavor and color.

7. Serve the tuna and white bean salad chilled or at room temperature.

Enjoy this refreshing and protein-packed Tuna and White Bean Salad! It's perfect for a quick and healthy lunch or dinner.

53. Grilled chicken with mango and avocado salsa

Ingredients:
- 4 boneless, skinless chicken breasts
- 2 ripe mangoes, diced
- 2 ripe avocados, diced
- 1 red bell pepper, diced
- 1/2 red onion, finely chopped
- 1/4 cup fresh cilantro, chopped
- Juice of 2 limes
- Salt and pepper to taste
- Olive oil

Instructions:
1. Preheat your grill to medium-high heat.

2. Season the chicken breasts with salt, pepper, and a drizzle of olive oil.

3. Grill the chicken breasts for about 6-7 minutes per side, or until they are cooked through and have nice grill marks. Cooking time may vary depending on the thickness of the chicken breasts. Ensure the internal temperature reaches 165°F (75°C).

4. While the chicken is grilling, prepare the salsa. In a mixing bowl, combine diced mangoes, diced avocados, diced red bell pepper, finely chopped red onion, chopped cilantro, and lime juice. Mix well and season with salt and pepper to taste.

5. Once the chicken is cooked, remove it from the grill and let it rest for a few minutes.

6. Serve the grilled chicken topped with the mango and avocado salsa.

This dish pairs wonderfully with rice, quinoa, or a fresh green salad. Enjoy your flavorful and nutritious meal!

54. Mediterranean chickpea salad

Ingredients:
- 2 cans (15 ounces each) chickpeas (garbanzo beans), rinsed and drained
- 1 English cucumber, diced
- 1 pint cherry tomatoes, halved
- 1/2 red onion, finely chopped
- 1/2 cup Kalamata olives, pitted and halved
- 1/4 cup fresh parsley, chopped
- 1/4 cup fresh mint leaves, chopped
- 4 ounces feta cheese, crumbled (optional)
- Juice of 2 lemons
- 3 tablespoons extra virgin olive oil
- 1 teaspoon dried oregano
- Salt and pepper to taste

Instructions:
1. In a large mixing bowl, combine the chickpeas, diced cucumber, halved cherry tomatoes, finely chopped red onion, halved Kalamata olives, chopped parsley, and chopped mint leaves. Toss gently to combine.

2. In a small bowl, whisk together the lemon juice, extra virgin olive oil, dried oregano, salt, and pepper to make the dressing.

3. Pour the dressing over the chickpea mixture and toss until everything is evenly coated.

4. If using, sprinkle crumbled feta cheese over the salad and gently toss to incorporate.

5. Taste and adjust seasoning if necessary.

6. Refrigerate the salad for at least 30 minutes before serving to allow the flavors to meld together.

7. Serve chilled as a side dish or as a light main course.

This Mediterranean chickpea salad is perfect for picnics, potlucks, or as a healthy lunch option. Enjoy its vibrant colors and delicious flavors!

55. Lentil and vegetable soup

Ingredients:
- 1 cup dried lentils (green or brown), rinsed and drained
- 1 onion, chopped
- 2 carrots, diced
- 2 celery stalks, diced
- 3 cloves garlic, minced
- 1 can (14.5 ounces) diced tomatoes
- 6 cups vegetable or chicken broth
- 1 teaspoon ground cumin
- 1 teaspoon ground coriander
- 1/2 teaspoon smoked paprika
- Salt and pepper to taste
- 2 tablespoons olive oil
- Fresh parsley or cilantro for garnish (optional)

Instructions:
1. In a large pot or Dutch oven, heat olive oil over medium heat.

2. Add chopped onion, diced carrots, and diced celery to the pot. Cook, stirring occasionally, until the vegetables are softened, about 5-7 minutes.

3. Add minced garlic to the pot and cook for another 1-2 minutes until fragrant.

4. Stir in the dried lentils, diced tomatoes (with their juices), vegetable or chicken broth, ground cumin, ground coriander, smoked paprika, salt, and pepper.

5. Bring the soup to a boil, then reduce the heat to low. Cover and simmer for about 25-30 minutes, or until the lentils are tender.

6. Once the lentils are cooked, taste the soup and adjust seasoning if necessary.

7. If you prefer a smoother texture, you can use an immersion blender to partially blend the soup, or transfer a portion of the soup to a blender and puree until smooth, then return it to the pot. Serve the lentil and vegetable soup hot, garnished with fresh parsley or cilantro if desired.

This soup is not only delicious and comforting but also rich in protein and fiber from the lentils and vegetables. Enjoy it as a wholesome meal on its own or with a slice of crusty bread for dipping!

56. Grilled shrimp and vegetable skewers

Ingredients:
- 1 pound large shrimp, peeled and deveined
- 2 bell peppers (any color), cut into chunks
- 1 red onion, cut into chunks
- 1 zucchini, sliced into rounds
- 1 yellow squash, sliced into rounds
- 8-10 cherry tomatoes
- 2 tablespoons olive oil
- 2 cloves garlic, minced
- 1 teaspoon smoked paprika
- 1 teaspoon dried oregano
- Salt and pepper to taste
- Wooden or metal skewers

Instructions:
1. If you're using wooden skewers, soak them in water for at least 30 minutes to prevent them from burning on the grill.

2. In a small bowl, whisk together olive oil, minced garlic, smoked paprika, dried oregano, salt, and pepper to make the marinade.

3. Place the shrimp in a separate bowl and pour half of the marinade over them. Toss to coat evenly. Let the shrimp marinate for about 15-20 minutes while you prepare the vegetables.

4. Preheat your grill to medium-high heat.

5. Thread the marinated shrimp, bell pepper chunks, red onion chunks, zucchini slices, yellow squash slices, and cherry tomatoes onto the skewers, alternating between ingredients.

6. Brush the vegetable skewers with the remaining marinade.

7. Grill the skewers for about 2-3 minutes per side, or until the shrimp are pink and opaque and the vegetables are tender and slightly charred.

8. Once cooked, remove the skewers from the grill and serve hot. Optionally, garnish with fresh chopped parsley or a squeeze of lemon juice before serving.

These grilled shrimp and vegetable skewers are not only delicious but also colorful and packed with nutrients. Serve them as a main course or as part of a larger barbecue spread.

57. Turkey and vegetable chili

Ingredients:
- 1 pound ground turkey
- 1 onion, diced
- 2 cloves garlic, minced
- 2 bell peppers (any color), diced
- 2 carrots, diced
- 2 celery stalks, diced
- 1 zucchini, diced
- 1 can (14.5 ounces) diced tomatoes
- 1 can (15 ounces) kidney beans, drained and rinsed
- 1 can (15 ounces) black beans, drained and rinsed
- 2 cups low-sodium chicken or vegetable broth
- 2 tablespoons tomato paste
- 2 tablespoons chili powder
- 1 teaspoon ground cumin
- 1 teaspoon smoked paprika
- Salt and pepper to taste
- Olive oil
- Optional toppings: shredded cheese, sour cream, chopped green onions, chopped cilantro, avocado slices

Instructions:

1. Heat a tablespoon of olive oil in a large pot or Dutch oven over medium heat.

2. Add diced onion to the pot and cook until softened, about 5 minutes.

3. Add minced garlic and cook for another minute until fragrant.

4. Add ground turkey to the pot and cook, breaking it apart with a spoon, until browned and cooked through.

5. Stir in diced bell peppers, carrots, celery, and zucchini. Cook for 5-7 minutes until the vegetables begin to soften.

6. Add diced tomatoes, kidney beans, black beans, chicken or vegetable broth, tomato paste, chili powder, ground cumin, smoked paprika, salt, and pepper to the pot. Stir to combine.

7. Bring the chili to a simmer, then reduce the heat to low. Cover and let it simmer for about 20-30 minutes, stirring occasionally, to allow the flavors to meld together and the vegetables to become tender.

8. Taste and adjust seasoning if necessary. Serve the turkey and vegetable chili hot, garnished with your choice of toppings such as shredded cheese, sour cream, chopped green onions, chopped cilantro, or avocado slices.

This turkey and vegetable chili is delicious, nutritious, and perfect for warming you up on a cold day. Enjoy it with some crusty bread or cornbread on the side for a complete meal!

58. Spinach and feta stuffed tomatoes

Ingredients:
- 4 large tomatoes
- 2 cups fresh spinach, chopped
- 1/2 cup crumbled feta cheese
- 2 cloves garlic, minced
- 2 tablespoons olive oil
- 1/4 teaspoon red pepper flakes (optional)
- Salt and pepper to taste
- 2 tablespoons grated Parmesan cheese (optional, for topping)
- Fresh basil leaves for garnish (optional)

Instructions:
1. Preheat your oven to 375°F (190°C).

2. Slice off the tops of the tomatoes and carefully scoop out the seeds and pulp from the center using a spoon, leaving a hollow shell. You can reserve the pulp for other recipes like sauces or soups.

3. In a skillet, heat olive oil over medium heat. Add minced garlic and red pepper flakes (if using) and cook for about 1 minute until fragrant.

4. Add chopped spinach to the skillet and cook, stirring occasionally, until wilted, about 2-3 minutes.

5. Remove the skillet from heat and let the spinach mixture cool slightly.

6. In a mixing bowl, combine the cooked spinach with crumbled feta cheese. Season with salt and pepper to taste.

7. Spoon the spinach and feta mixture into the hollowed-out tomatoes, pressing gently to fill them evenly.

8. Place the stuffed tomatoes in a baking dish. If desired, sprinkle grated Parmesan cheese over the tops of the stuffed tomatoes for an extra cheesy crust.

9. Bake in the preheated oven for about 20-25 minutes, or until the tomatoes are softened and the filling is heated through.

10. Once cooked, remove the stuffed tomatoes from the oven and let them cool slightly. Garnish with fresh basil leaves before serving, if desired.

These spinach and feta stuffed tomatoes make for an elegant and flavorful dish that's perfect for entertaining or as a side to accompany your main course. Enjoy the combination of juicy tomatoes, savory spinach, and tangy feta cheese!

59. Baked cod with tomatoes and basil

Ingredients:
- 4 cod fillets (about 6 ounces each)
- 2 cups cherry tomatoes, halved
- 1/4 cup fresh basil leaves, chopped
- 2 cloves garlic, minced
- 2 tablespoons olive oil
- 1 tablespoon balsamic vinegar
- Salt and pepper to taste
- Lemon wedges for serving (optional)

Instructions:
1. Preheat your oven to 400°F (200°C).

2. In a small bowl, combine halved cherry tomatoes, minced garlic, chopped basil leaves, olive oil, and balsamic vinegar. Season with salt and pepper to taste. Toss to coat the tomatoes evenly.

3. Season both sides of the cod fillets with salt and pepper.

4. Place the cod fillets in a baking dish, leaving some space between each fillet.

5. Spoon the tomato mixture over the top of the cod fillets, distributing it evenly.

6. Bake in the preheated oven for about 15-20 minutes, or until the cod is cooked through and flakes easily with a fork.

7. Once cooked, remove the baked cod from the oven and let it rest for a few minutes before serving.

8. Serve the baked cod with tomatoes and basil hot, garnished with additional fresh basil leaves and lemon wedges if desired.

This baked cod with tomatoes and basil is light, flavorful, and perfect for a healthy dinner option. Serve it with a side of steamed vegetables, rice, or crusty bread to complete the meal. Enjoy the vibrant flavors of the tomatoes and basil complementing the delicate taste of the cod!

60. Quinoa and roasted vegetable bowls

Ingredients:
- 1 cup quinoa, rinsed
- 2 cups water or vegetable broth
- 2 cups mixed vegetables (such as bell peppers, zucchini, eggplant, cherry tomatoes, carrots, broccoli, etc.), cut into bite-sized pieces
- 2 tablespoons olive oil
- 2 cloves garlic, minced
- 1 teaspoon dried herbs (such as thyme, rosemary, or Italian seasoning)
- Salt and pepper to taste
- Optional toppings: avocado slices, toasted nuts or seeds, crumbled feta cheese, chopped fresh herbs, balsamic glaze, etc.

Instructions:
1. Preheat your oven to 400°F (200°C).

2. In a medium saucepan, combine the quinoa and water or vegetable broth. Bring to a boil over medium-high heat, then reduce the heat to low, cover, and simmer for about 15-20 minutes, or until the quinoa is cooked and the liquid is absorbed. Remove from heat and let it sit covered for 5 minutes, then fluff with a fork.

3. While the quinoa is cooking, spread the mixed vegetables out on a baking sheet lined with parchment paper or aluminum foil.

4. In a small bowl, whisk together olive oil, minced garlic, dried herbs, salt, and pepper. Drizzle the mixture over the vegetables and toss to coat evenly.

5. Roast the vegetables in the preheated oven for about 20-25 minutes, or until they are tender and slightly caramelized, stirring halfway through cooking.

6. Once the quinoa and vegetables are ready, assemble the bowls by dividing the quinoa and roasted vegetables among serving bowls.

7. Add any desired toppings such as avocado slices, toasted nuts or seeds, crumbled feta cheese, or chopped fresh herbs.

8. Drizzle with balsamic glaze or a squeeze of lemon juice, if desired, for extra flavor. Serve the quinoa and roasted vegetable bowls hot and enjoy!

These quinoa and roasted vegetable bowls are versatile, nutritious, and perfect for meal prep. Feel free to customize them with your favorite vegetables, proteins, and toppings to create a delicious and balanced meal.

61. Grilled salmon with mango salsa

Ingredients:
- 4 salmon fillets (about 6 ounces each), skin-on or skinless
- 2 ripe mangoes, diced
- 1 red bell pepper, diced
- 1/2 red onion, finely chopped
- 1 jalapeño pepper, seeded and finely chopped (optional)
- 1/4 cup fresh cilantro, chopped
- Juice of 2 limes
- Salt and pepper to taste
- Olive oil
- Optional garnish: extra cilantro leaves, lime wedges

Instructions:
1. Preheat your grill to medium-high heat.

2. Season the salmon fillets with salt, pepper, and a drizzle of olive oil.

3. In a mixing bowl, combine diced mangoes, diced red bell pepper, finely chopped red onion, finely chopped jalapeño pepper (if using), chopped cilantro, and lime juice. Mix well and season with salt and pepper to taste.

4. Place the salmon fillets on the preheated grill, skin-side down if using skin-on fillets. Grill for about 4-5 minutes per side, or until the salmon is cooked through and easily flakes with a fork.

5. While the salmon is grilling, prepare the mango salsa. Taste and adjust seasoning if necessary.

6. Once the salmon is cooked, remove it from the grill and let it rest for a few minutes. Serve the grilled salmon hot, topped with the mango salsa.

7. Garnish with extra cilantro leaves and lime wedges if desired. Serve with your favorite side dishes such as rice, quinoa, or grilled vegetables.

This grilled salmon with mango salsa is not only delicious but also healthy and full of vibrant colors and flavors. Enjoy the combination of tender grilled salmon and juicy mango salsa for a delightful meal!

62. Turkey and vegetable lettuce wraps

Ingredients:
- 1 pound ground turkey
- 1 tablespoon olive oil
- 1 onion, diced
- 2 cloves garlic, minced
- 1 bell pepper, diced (any color)
- 1 zucchini, diced
- 1 carrot, grated
- 1/4 cup hoisin sauce
- 2 tablespoons soy sauce (or tamari for gluten-free option)
- 1 tablespoon rice vinegar
- 1 teaspoon sesame oil
- Salt and pepper to taste
- 1 head iceberg lettuce or butter lettuce, leaves separated
- Optional toppings: chopped green onions, chopped cilantro, chopped peanuts or cashews, sriracha sauce

Instructions:

1. Heat olive oil in a large skillet or wok over medium-high heat.

2. Add diced onion and minced garlic to the skillet and cook until softened and fragrant, about 2-3 minutes.

3. Add ground turkey to the skillet and cook, breaking it apart with a spoon, until browned and cooked through.

4. Stir in diced bell pepper, diced zucchini, and grated carrot. Cook for 3-4 minutes until the vegetables are tender-crisp.

5. In a small bowl, whisk together hoisin sauce, soy sauce, rice vinegar, sesame oil, salt, and pepper.

6. Pour the sauce mixture over the turkey and vegetable mixture in the skillet. Stir well to coat everything evenly.

7. Cook for another 2-3 minutes, stirring occasionally, until the sauce is heated through and the flavors are well combined. Taste and adjust seasoning if necessary.

8. To serve, spoon the turkey and vegetable mixture into individual lettuce leaves, using them as wraps.

9. Garnish with optional toppings such as chopped green onions, chopped cilantro, chopped peanuts or cashews, and a drizzle of sriracha sauce if desired. Roll up the lettuce leaves around the filling and enjoy immediately.

These turkey and vegetable lettuce wraps are not only delicious but also customizable to suit your taste preferences. They make for a flavorful and nutritious meal that's perfect for lunch or dinner. Enjoy the fresh crunch of lettuce paired with the savory turkey and vegetable filling!

63. Lentil and sweet potato curry

Ingredients:
- 1 teaspoon ground cumin
- 1 teaspoon ground coriander
- 1/2 teaspoon turmeric powder
- 1/4 teaspoon cayenne pepper
 (optional, for heat)
- Salt and pepper to taste
- 2 tablespoons olive oil
- Fresh cilantro leaves for
 garnish (optional)
- Cooked rice or
naan bread for serving
- 1 cup dried green or brown lentils, rinsed and drained
- 2 medium sweet potatoes, peeled and diced
- 1 onion, diced
- 2 cloves garlic, minced
- 1 tablespoon fresh ginger, minced
- 1 can (14 ounces) diced tomatoes
- 1 can (13.5 ounces) coconut milk
- 2 cups vegetable broth
- 2 tablespoons curry powder

Instructions:

1. Heat olive oil in a large pot or Dutch oven over medium heat.

2. Add diced onion to the pot and cook until softened, about 5 minutes.

3. Add minced garlic and minced ginger to the pot and cook for another 1-2 minutes until fragrant.

4. Stir in curry powder, ground cumin, ground coriander, turmeric powder, and cayenne pepper (if using). Cook for 1 minute, stirring constantly, until the spices are fragrant.

5. Add diced sweet potatoes, rinsed lentils, diced tomatoes (with their juices), coconut milk, and vegetable broth to the pot. Stir to combine.

6. Bring the mixture to a boil, then reduce the heat to low. Cover and simmer for about 20-25 minutes, or until the lentils and sweet potatoes are tender, stirring occasionally.

7. Once the lentils and sweet potatoes are cooked, taste the curry and adjust seasoning with salt and pepper if necessary.

8. If you prefer a thicker consistency, you can use an immersion blender to partially blend the curry, or transfer a portion of the curry to a blender and puree until smooth, then return it to the pot.

9. Serve the lentil and sweet potato curry hot, garnished with fresh cilantro leaves if desired. Enjoy the curry with cooked rice or naan bread for a complete meal.

64. Roasted Brussels sprouts with balsamic glaze

Ingredients:
- 1 pound Brussels sprouts, trimmed and halved
- 2 tablespoons olive oil
- Salt and pepper to taste
- 2-3 tablespoons balsamic glaze (store-bought or homemade*)

Instructions:
1. Preheat your oven to 400°F (200°C).

2. In a large mixing bowl, toss the halved Brussels sprouts with olive oil until they are evenly coated.

3. Season the Brussels sprouts with salt and pepper to taste.

4. Spread the Brussels sprouts out on a baking sheet lined with parchment paper or aluminum foil, making sure they are in a single layer and not too crowded.

5. Roast the Brussels sprouts in the preheated oven for about 20-25 minutes, or until they are golden brown and tender, stirring halfway through cooking for even browning.

6. Once the Brussels sprouts are roasted to your liking, remove them from the oven and transfer them to a serving dish.

7. Drizzle the roasted Brussels sprouts with balsamic glaze, using as much or as little as you prefer.

8. Toss the Brussels sprouts gently to coat them evenly with the balsamic glaze. Serve the roasted Brussels sprouts hot as a side dish.

To make homemade balsamic glaze:
- Pour 1 cup of balsamic vinegar into a small saucepan.
- Bring the vinegar to a boil over medium-high heat, then reduce the heat to low.
- Simmer the vinegar, stirring occasionally, until it reduces by half and thickens to a syrupy consistency, about 10-15 minutes.
- Remove the saucepan from the heat and let the balsamic glaze cool before using.

These roasted Brussels sprouts with balsamic glaze are flavorful, tender, and caramelized, with a touch of sweetness from the glaze. They make for a delicious side dish that pairs well with a variety of main courses. Enjoy!

65. Baked tilapia with tomatoes and olives

Ingredients:
- 4 tilapia fillets (about 6 ounces each)
- 2 cups cherry tomatoes, halved
- 1/2 cup Kalamata olives, pitted and halved
- 2 cloves garlic, minced
- 2 tablespoons olive oil
- 1 tablespoon balsamic vinegar
- 1 teaspoon dried oregano
- Salt and pepper to taste
- Lemon wedges for serving (optional)
- Fresh parsley for garnish (optional)

Instructions:
1. Preheat your oven to 400°F (200°C).

2. Place the tilapia fillets in a baking dish lined with parchment paper or aluminum foil. Season the fillets with salt and pepper to taste.

3. In a mixing bowl, combine halved cherry tomatoes, halved Kalamata olives, minced garlic, olive oil, balsamic vinegar, dried oregano, salt, and pepper. Toss to coat everything evenly.

4. Spoon the tomato and olive mixture over the tilapia fillets in the baking dish.

5. Bake in the preheated oven for about 15-20 minutes, or until the tilapia is cooked through and flakes easily with a fork.

6. Once cooked, remove the baked tilapia from the oven and let it rest for a few minutes.

7. Serve the tilapia hot, garnished with fresh parsley and lemon wedges if desired.

This baked tilapia with tomatoes and olives is light, flavorful, and perfect for a quick weeknight dinner. Enjoy the combination of tender tilapia, juicy tomatoes, and briny olives for a delicious meal!

66. Greek salad with grilled chicken

Ingredients:
- 2 boneless, skinless chicken breasts
- 1 tablespoon olive oil
- 1 teaspoon dried oregano
- Salt and pepper to taste
- 1 head romaine lettuce, chopped
- 1 cucumber, diced
- 1 bell pepper (any color), diced
- 1 pint cherry tomatoes, halved
- 1/2 red onion, thinly sliced
- 1/2 cup Kalamata olives, pitted
- 4 ounces feta cheese, crumbled
- Optional: 1/4 cup chopped fresh parsley or mint

For the dressing:
- 1/4 cup extra virgin olive oil
- 2 tablespoons red wine vinegar
- 1 teaspoon dried oregano
- 1 clove garlic, minced
- Salt and pepper to taste

Instructions:
1. Preheat your grill to medium-high heat.

2. Season the chicken breasts with olive oil, dried oregano, salt, and pepper.

3. Grill the chicken breasts for about 6-7 minutes per side, or until they are cooked through and have nice grill marks. Cooking time may vary depending on the thickness of the chicken breasts. Ensure the internal temperature reaches 165°F (75°C).

4. Once cooked, remove the chicken from the grill and let it rest for a few minutes before slicing.

5. While the chicken is grilling, prepare the salad ingredients. In a large mixing bowl, combine chopped romaine lettuce, diced cucumber, diced bell pepper, halved cherry tomatoes, thinly sliced red onion, Kalamata olives, and crumbled feta cheese. If using, add chopped fresh parsley or mint.

6. In a small bowl, whisk together extra virgin olive oil, red wine vinegar, dried oregano, minced garlic, salt, and pepper to make the dressing.

7. Pour the dressing over the salad and toss to coat everything evenly. Once the chicken has rested, slice it into thin strips.

8. Divide the Greek salad among serving plates and top each serving with sliced grilled chicken. Serve the Greek salad with grilled chicken immediately, and enjoy!

This Greek salad with grilled chicken is a satisfying and nutritious meal that's perfect for lunch or dinner. Enjoy the combination of crisp vegetables, tangy feta cheese, and flavorful grilled chicken!

67. Turkey and vegetable meatballs with zucchini noodles

Ingredients:
- For the meatballs: ground turkey, grated zucchini, grated carrot, onion, garlic, breadcrumbs, egg, parsley, oregano, salt, pepper, olive oil
- For the zucchini noodles: zucchini, olive oil, garlic, salt, pepper
- For serving: marinara sauce, Parmesan cheese, fresh basil or parsley (optional)

Instructions:
1. Mix meatball ingredients, shape into balls, and bake at 400°F (200°C) for 20-25 minutes.

2. Sauté garlic in olive oil, add zucchini noodles, and cook until tender.

3. Serve meatballs over zucchini noodles with marinara sauce.

4. Optional: garnish with Parmesan cheese and fresh herbs.

Enjoy this healthy and flavorful dish!

68. Roasted cauliflower and chickpea tacos

Ingredients:
- 1 head cauliflower, cut into small florets
- 1 can (15 ounces) chickpeas, drained and rinsed
- 2 tablespoons olive oil
- 1 teaspoon chili powder
- 1 teaspoon ground cumin
- 1/2 teaspoon smoked paprika
- 1/2 teaspoon garlic powder
- Salt and pepper to taste
- 8 small corn or flour tortillas
- Optional toppings: shredded lettuce, diced tomatoes, diced avocado, salsa, sour cream, chopped cilantro, lime wedges

Instructions:

1. Preheat your oven to 425°F (220°C).

2. In a large mixing bowl, toss the cauliflower florets and chickpeas with olive oil, chili powder, ground cumin, smoked paprika, garlic powder, salt, and pepper until evenly coated.

3. Spread the cauliflower and chickpea mixture out on a baking sheet lined with parchment paper or aluminum foil in a single layer.

4. Roast in the preheated oven for about 20-25 minutes, stirring halfway through cooking, until the cauliflower is tender and caramelized.

5. While the cauliflower and chickpeas are roasting, warm the tortillas in a dry skillet or microwave until heated through.

6. Once the cauliflower and chickpeas are roasted, remove them from the oven.

7. To assemble the tacos, divide the roasted cauliflower and chickpeas among the warmed tortillas.

8. Top each taco with your desired toppings such as shredded lettuce, diced tomatoes, diced avocado, salsa, sour cream, chopped cilantro, and a squeeze of lime juice. Serve the roasted cauliflower and chickpea tacos immediately, and enjoy!

These tacos are a delicious and satisfying vegetarian option that's packed with flavor and texture. Customize them with your favorite toppings and enjoy a tasty meal!

69. Grilled peach and arugula salad with balsamic dressing

Ingredients:
- 2 ripe peaches, halved and pitted
- 4 cups arugula leaves
- 1/4 cup crumbled goat cheese or feta cheese
- 1/4 cup chopped walnuts or pecans, toasted
- Balsamic glaze, for drizzling

For the balsamic dressing:
- 3 tablespoons extra virgin olive oil
- 2 tablespoons balsamic vinegar
- 1 teaspoon Dijon mustard
- 1 teaspoon honey or maple syrup (optional)
- Salt and pepper to taste

Instructions:
1. Preheat your grill or grill pan over medium-high heat.

2. In a small bowl, whisk together the ingredients for the balsamic dressing: olive oil, balsamic vinegar, Dijon mustard, honey or maple syrup (if using), salt, and pepper. Set aside.

3. Lightly brush the peach halves with olive oil to prevent sticking.

4. Place the peaches cut side down on the grill and cook for about 3-4 minutes, or until grill marks appear and the peaches are slightly softened.

5. Flip the peaches and grill for an additional 2-3 minutes on the other side. Remove from the grill and let them cool slightly.

6. In a large salad bowl, combine the arugula leaves, crumbled goat cheese or feta cheese, and toasted walnuts or pecans.

7. Slice the grilled peaches into wedges and add them to the salad bowl.

8. Drizzle the balsamic dressing over the salad and toss gently to coat everything evenly.

9. Divide the salad among serving plates.

10. Drizzle with balsamic glaze for an extra burst of flavor. Serve the grilled peach and arugula salad immediately, and enjoy!

This salad is perfect for summer gatherings or as a light and refreshing side dish. The combination of sweet grilled peaches, peppery arugula, tangy cheese, and crunchy nuts creates a delightful balance of flavors and textures.

70. Vegetarian stuffed peppers with quinoa and black beans

Ingredients:
- 4 large bell peppers, any color
- 1 cup cooked quinoa
- 1 can (15 ounces) black beans, drained and rinsed
- 1 cup corn kernels (fresh, frozen, or canned)
- 1 small onion, finely chopped
- 2 cloves garlic, minced
- 1 teaspoon ground cumin
- 1 teaspoon chili powder
- 1/2 teaspoon smoked paprika
- Salt and pepper to taste
- 1 cup shredded cheese (such as cheddar, Monterey Jack, or Mexican blend)
- Fresh cilantro or parsley for garnish (optional)

Instructions:
1. Preheat your oven to 375°F (190°C). Grease a baking dish large enough to hold the peppers.

2. Cut the tops off the bell peppers and remove the seeds and membranes. Place the peppers upright in the prepared baking dish.

3. In a large mixing bowl, combine cooked quinoa, black beans, corn kernels, chopped onion, minced garlic, ground cumin, chili powder, smoked paprika, salt, and pepper. Mix well to combine.

4. Spoon the quinoa and black bean mixture into the hollowed-out bell peppers, pressing down gently to pack the filling.

5. Cover the baking dish with aluminum foil and bake in the preheated oven for 25-30 minutes, or until the peppers are tender.

6. Remove the foil from the baking dish and sprinkle the shredded cheese over the stuffed peppers.

7. Return the baking dish to the oven and bake for an additional 5-10 minutes, or until the cheese is melted and bubbly.

8. Once cooked, remove the stuffed peppers from the oven and let them cool slightly before serving. Garnish with fresh cilantro or parsley, if desired, before serving

71. Baked salmon with pineapple salsa

Ingredients:
- 4 salmon fillets (about 6 ounces each)
- Salt and pepper to taste
- Olive oil
- 2 cups diced pineapple
- 1/2 red onion, finely chopped
- 1 red bell pepper, diced
- 1 jalapeño pepper, seeded and finely chopped
- Juice of 1 lime
- 2 tablespoons chopped fresh cilantro
- Salt and pepper to taste

Instructions:
1. Preheat your oven to 375°F (190°C).

2. Place the salmon fillets on a baking sheet lined with parchment paper or aluminum foil. Season them with salt, pepper, and a drizzle of olive oil.

3. Bake the salmon in the preheated oven for about 12-15 minutes, or until the salmon is cooked through and flakes easily with a fork.

4. While the salmon is baking, prepare the pineapple salsa. In a mixing bowl, combine diced pineapple, finely chopped red onion, diced red bell pepper, finely chopped jalapeño pepper, lime juice, chopped cilantro, salt, and pepper. Mix well to combine.

5. Once the salmon is cooked, remove it from the oven and let it rest for a few minutes.

6. Serve the baked salmon hot, topped with the pineapple salsa.

7. Enjoy the flavorful combination of tender salmon and sweet-spicy pineapple salsa!

This baked salmon with pineapple salsa is a light, healthy, and vibrant dish that's perfect for summer. It's sure to impress your family and friends with its delicious flavors!

72. Tuna and white bean salad

Ingredients:
- 2 cans (5 ounces each) tuna, drained
- 1 can (15 ounces) white beans (such as cannellini or Great Northern), drained and rinsed
- 1/2 red onion, finely chopped
- 1 celery stalk, finely chopped
- 1/4 cup chopped fresh parsley
- 2 tablespoons capers, drained
- Juice of 1 lemon
- 2 tablespoons extra virgin olive oil
- Salt and pepper to taste
- Optional: sliced cherry tomatoes, sliced cucumber, chopped bell pepper, olives

Instructions:

1. In a large mixing bowl, combine the drained tuna, white beans, finely chopped red onion, finely chopped celery, chopped fresh parsley, and capers.

2. Drizzle the lemon juice and extra virgin olive oil over the salad ingredients.

3. Season with salt and pepper to taste.

4. Gently toss everything together until well combined.

5. Taste and adjust seasoning if necessary.

6. If desired, add optional ingredients such as sliced cherry tomatoes, sliced cucumber, chopped bell pepper, or olives.

7. Serve the tuna and white bean salad chilled or at room temperature.

8. Enjoy as a light and satisfying meal or as a side dish!

This tuna and white bean salad is quick and easy to make, and it's packed with protein and fiber. It's perfect for a quick lunch or a light dinner, and you can customize it with your favorite ingredients!

73. Grilled chicken with mango and avocado salsa

Ingredients:
- 4 boneless, skinless chicken breasts
- Salt and pepper to taste
- 1 tablespoon olive oil
- 1 teaspoon ground cumin
- 1 teaspoon chili powder
- 1/2 teaspoon garlic powder
- 1 ripe mango, peeled, pitted, and diced
- 1 ripe avocado, peeled, pitted, and diced
- 1/4 cup red onion, finely chopped
- 1/4 cup fresh cilantro, chopped
- Juice of 1 lime
- Salt and pepper to taste

Instructions:
1. Preheat your grill to medium-high heat.

2. Season the chicken breasts with salt, pepper, ground cumin, chili powder, and garlic powder. Drizzle with olive oil and rub the seasonings evenly over the chicken.

3. Grill the chicken breasts for about 6-8 minutes per side, or until they are cooked through and have grill marks. Cooking time may vary depending on the thickness of the chicken breasts. Ensure the internal temperature reaches 165°F (75°C).

4. While the chicken is grilling, prepare the mango and avocado salsa. In a mixing bowl, combine diced mango, diced avocado, finely chopped red onion, chopped fresh cilantro, and lime juice. Season with salt and pepper to taste. Gently toss to combine.

5. Once the chicken is cooked, remove it from the grill and let it rest for a few minutes.

6. Serve the grilled chicken hot, topped with mango and avocado salsa.

7. Enjoy the flavorful combination of tender grilled chicken with the refreshing sweetness of mango and creamy avocado!

This grilled chicken with mango and avocado salsa is perfect for a light and vibrant summer meal. It's easy to make and bursting with fresh flavors!

74. Roasted cauliflower and chickpea salad

Ingredients:
- 1 head cauliflower, cut into florets
- 1 can (15 ounces) chickpeas, drained and rinsed
- 2 tablespoons olive oil
- 1 teaspoon ground cumin
- 1 teaspoon paprika
- 1/2 teaspoon garlic powder
- Salt and pepper to taste
- 4 cups mixed greens (such as spinach, arugula, or kale)
- 1/4 cup dried cranberries or raisins
- 1/4 cup chopped fresh parsley
- 2 tablespoons lemon juice
- Optional: crumbled feta cheese, toasted nuts or seeds

Instructions:
1. Preheat your oven to 400°F (200°C).

2. In a large mixing bowl, toss the cauliflower florets and chickpeas with olive oil, ground cumin, paprika, garlic powder, salt, and pepper until evenly coated.

3. Spread the cauliflower and chickpea mixture out on a baking sheet lined with parchment paper or aluminum foil in a single layer.

4. Roast in the preheated oven for about 25-30 minutes, or until the cauliflower is tender and golden brown, stirring halfway through cooking for even browning.

5. While the cauliflower and chickpeas are roasting, prepare the salad. In a large salad bowl, combine the mixed greens, dried cranberries or raisins, and chopped fresh parsley.

6. Once the cauliflower and chickpeas are roasted, remove them from the oven and let them cool slightly.

7. Add the roasted cauliflower and chickpeas to the salad bowl with the mixed greens. Drizzle the lemon juice over the salad and toss gently to combine.

8. If desired, top the salad with crumbled feta cheese and toasted nuts or seeds for extra flavor and texture. Serve the roasted cauliflower and chickpea salad immediately, and enjoy!

This salad is nutritious, flavorful, and satisfying. It's perfect for a light lunch or dinner and can be easily customized with your favorite toppings and dressings!

75. Lentil and vegetable soup

Ingredients:
- 1 cup dried green or brown lentils, rinsed and drained
- 4 cups vegetable broth
- 1 onion, diced
- 2 carrots, diced
- 2 celery stalks, diced
- 2 cloves garlic, minced
- 1 can (14 ounces) diced tomatoes
- 1 teaspoon dried thyme
- 1 teaspoon dried oregano
- Salt and pepper to taste
- 2 cups chopped spinach or kale
- 2 tablespoons olive oil
- Optional garnish: chopped fresh parsley, grated Parmesan cheese

Instructions:

1. In a large pot or Dutch oven, heat olive oil over medium heat.

2. Add diced onion, carrots, and celery to the pot. Cook, stirring occasionally, until the vegetables are softened, about 5-7 minutes.

3. Add minced garlic to the pot and cook for another 1-2 minutes until fragrant.

4. Stir in dried thyme and dried oregano, and cook for 1 minute, stirring constantly.

5. Add rinsed lentils, diced tomatoes (with their juices), and vegetable broth to the pot. Stir to combine.

6. Bring the soup to a boil, then reduce the heat to low. Cover and simmer for about 20-25 minutes, or until the lentils are tender.

7. Once the lentils are cooked, stir in chopped spinach or kale and cook for an additional 3-5 minutes until wilted.

8. Taste the soup and adjust seasoning with salt and pepper if necessary.

9. Ladle the lentil and vegetable soup into bowls. Optionally, garnish with chopped fresh parsley and grated Parmesan cheese. Serve the soup hot, and enjoy!

This lentil and vegetable soup is hearty, nutritious, and perfect for a comforting meal. It's packed with fiber, vitamins, and minerals, making it a wholesome option for lunch or dinner.

76. Grilled shrimp and vegetable skewers

Ingredients:
- 1 pound large shrimp, peeled and deveined
- 2 bell peppers (any color), cut into chunks
- 1 red onion, cut into chunks
- 1 zucchini, sliced
- 1 yellow squash, sliced
- Cherry tomatoes
- Olive oil
- Salt and pepper to taste
- Optional: lemon wedges, chopped fresh herbs (such as parsley or basil) for garnish

Instructions:

1. If using wooden skewers, soak them in water for about 30 minutes to prevent them from burning on the grill.

2. Preheat your grill to medium-high heat.

3. Thread the shrimp and vegetables onto skewers, alternating between the shrimp and vegetables.

4. Brush the skewers with olive oil and season with salt and pepper to taste.

5. Place the skewers on the preheated grill and cook for about 2-3 minutes per side, or until the shrimp is pink and opaque and the vegetables are tender and lightly charred.

6. Once cooked, remove the skewers from the grill and transfer them to a serving platter.

7. Optionally, garnish with lemon wedges and chopped fresh herbs before serving.

8. Serve the grilled shrimp and vegetable skewers hot, and enjoy!

These skewers are perfect for a summer barbecue or a quick and healthy weeknight meal. They're versatile and can be customized with your favorite vegetables and seasonings. Enjoy the delicious combination of tender shrimp and grilled vegetables!

77. Turkey and vegetable chili

Ingredients:
- 1 pound ground turkey
- 1 tablespoon olive oil
- 1 onion, diced
- 2 cloves garlic, minced
- 1 bell pepper (any color), diced
- 1 zucchini, diced
- 1 carrot, diced
- 1 can (15 ounces) diced tomatoes
- 1 can (15 ounces) kidney beans, drained and rinsed
- 2 cups chicken or vegetable broth
- 2 tablespoons tomato paste
- 2 teaspoons chili powder
- 1 teaspoon ground cumin
- 1 teaspoon paprika
- Salt and pepper to taste
- Optional toppings: shredded cheese, chopped green onions, diced avocado, sour cream, chopped cilantro

Instructions:

1. Heat olive oil in a large pot or Dutch oven over medium heat.

2. Add diced onion and minced garlic to the pot and cook until softened and fragrant, about 2-3 minutes.

3. Add ground turkey to the pot and cook, breaking it apart with a spoon, until browned and cooked through.

4. Stir in diced bell pepper, diced zucchini, and diced carrot. Cook for 3-4 minutes until the vegetables are tender-crisp.

5. Add diced tomatoes, drained kidney beans, chicken or vegetable broth, tomato paste, chili powder, ground cumin, paprika, salt, and pepper to the pot. Stir to combine.

6. Bring the chili to a boil, then reduce the heat to low. Cover and simmer for about 20-25 minutes, stirring occasionally.

7. Taste the chili and adjust seasoning if necessary.

8. Serve the turkey and vegetable chili hot, topped with optional toppings such as shredded cheese, chopped green onions, diced avocado, sour cream, and chopped cilantro.

9. Enjoy the comforting and flavorful turkey and vegetable chili!

This chili is packed with protein and fiber from the turkey, beans, and vegetables, making it a nutritious and satisfying meal. It's perfect for chilly evenings or for feeding a crowd at gatherings.

78. Spinach and feta stuffed mushrooms

Ingredients:
- 16 large mushrooms, cleaned with stems removed
- 2 tablespoons olive oil
- 2 cloves garlic, minced
- 4 cups fresh spinach, chopped
- 1/2 cup crumbled feta cheese
- 1/4 cup grated Parmesan cheese
- Salt and pepper to taste
- Optional: chopped fresh parsley for garnish

Instructions:
1. Preheat your oven to 375°F (190°C).

2. In a large skillet, heat olive oil over medium heat.

3. Add minced garlic to the skillet and cook for about 1 minute until fragrant.

4. Add chopped spinach to the skillet and cook, stirring occasionally, until wilted, about 2-3 minutes.

5. Remove the skillet from the heat and let the spinach cool slightly.

6. In a mixing bowl, combine the cooked spinach, crumbled feta cheese, grated Parmesan cheese, salt, and pepper. Mix well to combine.

7. Spoon the spinach and feta mixture into the mushroom caps, pressing down gently to fill them evenly.

8. Place the stuffed mushrooms on a baking sheet lined with parchment paper or aluminum foil.

9. Bake in the preheated oven for about 15-20 minutes, or until the mushrooms are tender and the filling is heated through.

10. Once cooked, remove the stuffed mushrooms from the oven and let them cool slightly. Garnish with chopped fresh parsley, if desired, before serving.

12. Serve the spinach and feta stuffed mushrooms warm as a delicious appetizer or side dish.

79. Baked cod with tomatoes and basil

Ingredients:
- 4 cod fillets (about 6 ounces each)
- Salt and pepper to taste
- 2 tablespoons olive oil
- 2 cloves garlic, minced
- 1 pint cherry tomatoes, halved
- 1/4 cup chopped fresh basil
- 2 tablespoons balsamic glaze
- Lemon wedges for serving (optional)

Instructions:
1. Preheat your oven to 400°F (200°C).

2. Season the cod fillets with salt and pepper to taste.

3. In a large oven-safe skillet, heat olive oil over medium heat.

4. Add minced garlic to the skillet and cook for about 1 minute until fragrant.

5. Add cherry tomatoes to the skillet and cook for 2-3 minutes until they start to soften.

6. Remove the skillet from the heat and stir in chopped fresh basil.

7. Place the seasoned cod fillets on top of the tomato mixture in the skillet.

8. Drizzle the cod fillets with balsamic glaze.

9. Transfer the skillet to the preheated oven and bake for about 12-15 minutes, or until the cod is cooked through and flakes easily with a fork.

10. Once cooked, remove the skillet from the oven.

11. Serve the baked cod with tomatoes and basil hot, garnished with lemon wedges if desired.

This baked cod with tomatoes and basil is a light and delicious dish that's perfect for a quick and healthy weeknight dinner. The combination of tender cod, juicy tomatoes, and fragrant basil creates a flavorful meal that's sure to please!

80. Quinoa and roasted vegetable bowls

Ingredients:
- 1 cup quinoa, rinsed
- 2 cups water or vegetable broth
- 1 small sweet potato, peeled and diced
- 1 red bell pepper, diced
- 1 zucchini, diced
- 1 small red onion, diced
- 2 tablespoons olive oil
- Salt and pepper to taste
- 1 teaspoon ground cumin
- 1 teaspoon smoked paprika
- 1 avocado, sliced
- 1/4 cup crumbled feta cheese or goat cheese (optional)
- Fresh cilantro or parsley for garnish (optional)
- Optional dressing: balsamic vinaigrette, tahini dressing, or your favorite dressing

Instructions:

1. Preheat your oven to 400°F (200°C).

2. In a saucepan, combine quinoa and water or vegetable broth. Bring to a boil, then reduce the heat to low, cover, and simmer for 15-20 minutes, or until the quinoa is cooked and the liquid is absorbed.

3. While the quinoa is cooking, spread the diced sweet potato, red bell pepper, zucchini, and red onion on a baking sheet lined with parchment paper or aluminum foil.

4. Drizzle the vegetables with olive oil and sprinkle with salt, pepper, ground cumin, and smoked paprika. Toss to coat evenly.

5. Roast the vegetables in the preheated oven for 20-25 minutes, or until they are tender and lightly browned, stirring halfway through cooking.

6. Once the quinoa and vegetables are cooked, assemble the bowls. Divide the cooked quinoa among serving bowls and top with roasted vegetables.

7. Add sliced avocado on top of the bowls. If desired, sprinkle with crumbled feta cheese or goat cheese.

8. Garnish with fresh cilantro or parsley, if using.

9. Drizzle with your favorite dressing, if desired, or serve the bowls as is.

10. Serve the quinoa and roasted vegetable bowls hot, and enjoy!

These bowls are customizable, nutritious, and perfect for meal prep. Feel free to add other toppings such as toasted nuts or seeds, grilled tofu or chicken, or a squeeze of lime juice for extra flavor.

81. Grilled salmon with mango salsa

Ingredients:
- 4 salmon fillets (about 6 ounces each), skin-on
- Salt and pepper to taste
- Olive oil

For the mango salsa:
- 2 ripe mangoes, peeled, pitted, and diced
- 1/2 red onion, finely chopped
- 1 red bell pepper, diced
- 1 jalapeño pepper, seeded and finely chopped
- Juice of 1 lime
- 2 tablespoons chopped fresh cilantro
- Salt and pepper to taste

Instructions:
1. Preheat your grill to medium-high heat.

2. Season the salmon fillets with salt and pepper to taste. Drizzle with olive oil and rub to coat evenly.

3. Place the salmon fillets on the preheated grill, skin-side down. Grill for about 4-5 minutes per side, or until the salmon is cooked through and flakes easily with a fork.

4. While the salmon is grilling, prepare the mango salsa. In a mixing bowl, combine diced mangoes, finely chopped red onion, diced red bell pepper, finely chopped jalapeño pepper, lime juice, chopped fresh cilantro, salt, and pepper. Mix well to combine.

5. Once the salmon is cooked, remove it from the grill and let it rest for a few minutes.

6. Serve the grilled salmon hot, topped with mango salsa.

7. Enjoy the delicious combination of tender grilled salmon and fresh, vibrant mango salsa!

This grilled salmon with mango salsa is perfect for a light and refreshing summer meal. The sweet and tangy salsa complements the rich flavor of the salmon beautifully.

82. Turkey and vegetable lettuce wraps

Ingredients:
- 1 pound ground turkey
- 2 tablespoons olive oil
- 1 small onion, finely chopped
- 2 cloves garlic, minced
- 1 bell pepper (any color), finely chopped
- 1 carrot, grated
- 1/2 cup chopped mushrooms
- 1/4 cup hoisin sauce
- 2 tablespoons soy sauce (or tamari for gluten-free)
- 1 teaspoon sesame oil
- Salt and pepper to taste
- 1 head iceberg or butter lettuce, leaves separated
- Optional toppings: sliced green onions, chopped cilantro, chopped peanuts

Instructions:
1. Heat olive oil in a large skillet over medium heat.

2. Add chopped onion and minced garlic to the skillet. Cook until softened and fragrant, about 2-3 minutes.

3. Add ground turkey to the skillet and cook, breaking it apart with a spoon, until browned and cooked through.

4. Stir in chopped bell pepper, grated carrot, and chopped mushrooms. Cook for 3-4 minutes until the vegetables are tender-crisp.

5. In a small bowl, whisk together hoisin sauce, soy sauce, and sesame oil. Pour the sauce over the turkey and vegetable mixture in the skillet. Stir to combine.

6. Season with salt and pepper to taste. Cook for another 1-2 minutes until everything is heated through.

7. To serve, spoon the turkey and vegetable mixture onto individual lettuce leaves.

8. Optionally, top with sliced green onions, chopped cilantro, and chopped peanuts for extra flavor and texture. Roll up the lettuce leaves like tacos or wraps, and enjoy!

These turkey and vegetable lettuce wraps are easy to make, customizable, and perfect for a quick and healthy meal. They're packed with protein and veggies, making them a satisfying option for lunch or dinner.

83. Lentil and sweet potato stew

Ingredients:
- 1 cup dried green or brown lentils, rinsed and drained
- 2 large sweet potatoes, peeled and diced
- 1 onion, diced
- 2 cloves garlic, minced
- 1 bell pepper (any color), diced
- 1 can (14 ounces) diced tomatoes
- 4 cups vegetable broth
- 2 teaspoons ground cumin
- 1 teaspoon ground coriander
- 1 teaspoon smoked paprika
- Salt and pepper to taste
- 2 cups chopped kale or spinach
- Optional toppings: chopped fresh cilantro, Greek yogurt, lime wedges

Instructions:

1. In a large pot or Dutch oven, heat olive oil over medium heat.

2. Add diced onion and minced garlic to the pot. Cook until softened and fragrant, about 2-3 minutes.

3. Add diced sweet potatoes and diced bell pepper to the pot. Cook for another 5 minutes, stirring occasionally.

4. Stir in dried lentils, diced tomatoes (with their juices), vegetable broth, ground cumin, ground coriander, smoked paprika, salt, and pepper. Mix well to combine.

5. Bring the stew to a boil, then reduce the heat to low. Cover and simmer for about 20-25 minutes, or until the lentils and sweet potatoes are tender.

6. Once the lentils and sweet potatoes are cooked, stir in chopped kale or spinach. Cook for an additional 3-5 minutes until the greens are wilted.

7. Taste the stew and adjust seasoning with salt and pepper if necessary.

8. Serve the lentil and sweet potato stew hot, garnished with optional toppings such as chopped fresh cilantro, a dollop of Greek yogurt, or a squeeze of lime juice. Enjoy this comforting and nutritious stew!

This lentil and sweet potato stew is rich in fiber, vitamins, and minerals, making it a satisfying and wholesome meal option. It's perfect for chilly days and can be easily customized with your favorite herbs and spices.

84. Roasted Brussels sprouts with balsamic glaze

Ingredients:
- 1 pound Brussels sprouts, trimmed and halved
- 2 tablespoons olive oil
- Salt and pepper to taste
- 2 tablespoons balsamic glaze (store-bought or homemade*)

Instructions:
1. Preheat your oven to 400°F (200°C).

2. Place the trimmed and halved Brussels sprouts on a baking sheet lined with parchment paper or aluminum foil.

3. Drizzle the Brussels sprouts with olive oil and toss to coat evenly. Season with salt and pepper to taste.

4. Spread the Brussels sprouts out in a single layer on the baking sheet.

5. Roast in the preheated oven for about 20-25 minutes, or until the Brussels sprouts are tender and caramelized, stirring halfway through cooking for even browning.

6. Once the Brussels sprouts are roasted to your liking, remove them from the oven and transfer them to a serving dish.

7. Drizzle the roasted Brussels sprouts with balsamic glaze. Toss gently to coat the Brussels sprouts in the glaze.

9. Serve the roasted Brussels sprouts with balsamic glaze hot as a delicious side dish or appetizer.

Enjoy the crispy, caramelized exterior and tender interior of the Brussels sprouts, paired with the sweet and tangy flavor of the balsamic glaze!

To make homemade balsamic glaze:
   - In a small saucepan, bring 1 cup of balsamic vinegar to a boil over medium-high heat.

   - Reduce the heat to low and simmer for about 10-15 minutes, or until the vinegar has thickened and reduced by half, stirring occasionally.

   - Remove the saucepan from the heat and let the balsamic glaze cool before using. It will continue to thicken as it cools.

85. Baked tilapia with tomatoes and olives

Ingredients:
- 4 tilapia fillets (about 6 ounces each)
- Salt and pepper to taste
- 2 tablespoons olive oil
- 2 cloves garlic, minced
- 1 pint cherry tomatoes, halved
- 1/4 cup sliced Kalamata olives
- 2 tablespoons chopped fresh parsley
- 1 lemon, sliced
- Optional: crumbled feta cheese for garnish

Instructions:
1. Preheat your oven to 375°F (190°C).

2. Season the tilapia fillets with salt and pepper to taste.

3. In a large oven-safe skillet or baking dish, heat olive oil over medium heat.

4. Add minced garlic to the skillet and cook for about 1 minute until fragrant.

5. Add cherry tomatoes and sliced Kalamata olives to the skillet. Cook for 2-3 minutes until the tomatoes start to soften.

6. Remove the skillet from the heat and stir in chopped fresh parsley.

7. Place the seasoned tilapia fillets on top of the tomato and olive mixture in the skillet.

8. Arrange lemon slices on top of the tilapia fillets.

9. Transfer the skillet to the preheated oven and bake for about 15-20 minutes, or until the tilapia is cooked through and flakes easily with a fork.

10. Once cooked, remove the skillet from the oven.

11. Optionally, garnish the baked tilapia with crumbled feta cheese before serving. Serve the baked tilapia with tomatoes and olives hot, and enjoy!

This baked tilapia with tomatoes and olives is a flavorful and easy-to-make dish that's perfect for a quick and healthy weeknight dinner. The combination of juicy tomatoes, briny olives, and fresh parsley complements the mild flavor of the tilapia beautifully.

86. Greek salad with grilled chicken

Ingredients:
- 2 boneless, skinless chicken breasts
- Salt and pepper to taste
- 2 tablespoons olive oil
- 1 teaspoon dried oregano
- 1 teaspoon dried thyme
- 1 teaspoon garlic powder
- 1 teaspoon onion powder
- 1 cucumber, diced
- 1 pint cherry tomatoes, halved
- 1/2 red onion, thinly sliced
- 1/2 cup Kalamata olives, pitted
- 1/2 cup crumbled feta cheese
- 1/4 cup chopped fresh parsley
- Juice of 1 lemon
- 2 tablespoons red wine vinegar
- 3 tablespoons extra virgin olive oil
- Salt and pepper to taste
- Optional: pita bread or crusty bread for serving

Instructions:

1. Preheat your grill to medium-high heat.

2. Season the chicken breasts with salt, pepper, dried oregano, dried thyme, garlic powder, and onion powder. Drizzle with olive oil and rub the seasonings evenly over the chicken.

3. Grill the chicken breasts for about 6-8 minutes per side, or until they are cooked through and have grill marks. Cooking time may vary depending on the thickness of the chicken breasts. Ensure the internal temperature reaches 165°F (75°C).

4. While the chicken is grilling, prepare the Greek salad. In a large mixing bowl, combine diced cucumber, halved cherry tomatoes, thinly sliced red onion, pitted Kalamata olives, crumbled feta cheese, and chopped fresh parsley.

5. In a small bowl, whisk together lemon juice, red wine vinegar, and extra virgin olive oil to make the dressing. Season with salt and pepper to taste.

6. Once the chicken is cooked, remove it from the grill and let it rest for a few minutes.

7. Slice the grilled chicken breasts into strips. Add the sliced grilled chicken to the Greek salad.

8. Drizzle the salad with the prepared dressing and toss gently to combine. Serve the Greek salad with grilled chicken immediately, and enjoy!

This Greek salad with grilled chicken is fresh, flavorful, and satisfying. It's perfect for a light and healthy meal, especially on warm summer days. Serve it with pita bread or crusty bread for a complete and delicious meal!

87. Turkey and vegetable meatballs with zucchini noodles

Ingredients:
- 1 lb ground turkey
- 1/2 cup breadcrumbs
- 1/4 cup each: grated Parmesan, chopped onion, grated carrot, chopped bell pepper
- 2 cloves garlic, minced
- 1 tsp each: dried oregano, dried basil
- Salt and pepper
- Olive oil
- 4 medium zucchini, spiralized
- Optional: chopped fresh parsley or basil

Instructions:
1. Preheat oven to 400°F (200°C).

2. Mix turkey, breadcrumbs, Parmesan, onion, carrot, bell pepper, garlic, oregano, basil, salt, and pepper. Form into meatballs.

3. Brown meatballs in olive oil in a skillet, then bake for 10-12 mins.

4. Sauté garlic in olive oil, add zucchini noodles, cook until tender.

5. Serve meatballs over zucchini noodles, garnish with parsley or basil if desired.

Enjoy this quick and healthy turkey and vegetable meatball dish with zucchini noodles!

88. Roasted cauliflower and chickpea tacos

Ingredients:
- 1 head cauliflower, cut into florets
- 1 can (15 ounces) chickpeas, drained and rinsed
- 2 tablespoons olive oil
- 1 teaspoon chili powder
- 1/2 teaspoon cumin
- 1/2 teaspoon paprika
- 1/4 teaspoon garlic powder
- Salt and pepper to taste
- 8 small tortillas (corn or flour)
- Toppings: shredded lettuce, diced tomatoes, sliced avocado, chopped cilantro, lime wedges, salsa, Greek yogurt or sour cream

Instructions:
1. Preheat your oven to 400°F (200°C).

2. In a large mixing bowl, toss cauliflower florets and chickpeas with olive oil, chili powder, cumin, paprika, garlic powder, salt, and pepper until evenly coated.

3. Spread the cauliflower and chickpea mixture out on a baking sheet lined with parchment paper or aluminum foil in a single layer.

4. Roast in the preheated oven for about 25-30 minutes, or until the cauliflower is tender and chickpeas are crispy, stirring halfway through cooking for even browning.

5. Warm tortillas according to package instructions.

6. Once the cauliflower and chickpeas are roasted, assemble the tacos by filling each tortilla with the roasted cauliflower and chickpea mixture.

7. Top the tacos with shredded lettuce, diced tomatoes, sliced avocado, chopped cilantro, and any other desired toppings.

8. Serve the roasted cauliflower and chickpea tacos with lime wedges, salsa, Greek yogurt or sour cream on the side. Enjoy the flavorful and satisfying vegetarian tacos!

These roasted cauliflower and chickpea tacos are packed with flavor and texture, making them a delicious and nutritious meal option for vegetarians and meat-lovers alike. Customize the toppings to suit your taste preferences and enjoy!

89. Grilled peach and arugula salad with balsamic dressing

Ingredients:
- 2 ripe peaches, halved and pitted
- 4 cups baby arugula
- 1/4 cup crumbled goat cheese or feta cheese
- 1/4 cup chopped walnuts or pecans, toasted
- Balsamic glaze for drizzling

For the balsamic dressing:
- 3 tablespoons extra virgin olive oil
- 2 tablespoons balsamic vinegar
- 1 teaspoon honey or maple syrup
- Salt and pepper to taste

Instructions:

1. Preheat your grill to medium-high heat.

2. In a small bowl, whisk together the ingredients for the balsamic dressing: extra virgin olive oil, balsamic vinegar, honey or maple syrup, salt, and pepper. Set aside.

3. Place the peach halves on the preheated grill, cut side down. Grill for about 3-4 minutes, or until grill marks form and the peaches are slightly softened.

4. Remove the grilled peaches from the grill and let them cool slightly.

5. In a large mixing bowl, combine baby arugula, crumbled goat cheese or feta cheese, and toasted walnuts or pecans.

6. Slice the grilled peaches and add them to the salad.

7. Drizzle the balsamic dressing over the salad and toss gently to coat.

8. Divide the salad onto plates or a serving platter.

9. Drizzle with balsamic glaze for extra flavor and presentation.

10. Serve the grilled peach and arugula salad immediately, and enjoy!

This salad is a perfect balance of sweet, savory, and tangy flavors, with the grilled peaches adding a delicious caramelized touch. It's a light and refreshing dish that's perfect for summer gatherings or as a side dish for grilled meats.

90. Vegetarian chili with sweet potatoes and black beans

Ingredients:
- 2 tablespoons olive oil
- 1 onion, diced
- 2 cloves garlic, minced
- 1 bell pepper (any color), diced
- 2 medium sweet potatoes,
 peeled and diced
- 1 can (15 ounces) black beans,
drained and rinsed
- 1 can (15 ounces) diced tomatoes

- 2 cups vegetable broth
- 1 tablespoon chili powder
- 1 teaspoon ground cumin
- 1/2 teaspoon smoked paprika
- Salt and pepper to taste
- Optional toppings: chopped fresh cilantro, diced avocado, shredded cheese, sour cream, lime wedges

Instructions:

1. Heat olive oil in a large pot or Dutch oven over medium heat.

2. Add diced onion and minced garlic to the pot. Cook until softened and fragrant, about 2-3 minutes.

3. Add diced bell pepper and diced sweet potatoes to the pot. Cook for another 5 minutes, stirring occasionally.

4. Stir in drained and rinsed black beans, diced tomatoes (with their juices), vegetable broth, chili powder, ground cumin, smoked paprika, salt, and pepper. Mix well to combine.

5. Bring the chili to a boil, then reduce the heat to low. Cover and simmer for about 20-25 minutes, or until the sweet potatoes are tender, stirring occasionally.

6. Taste the chili and adjust seasoning with salt and pepper if necessary.

7. Once the sweet potatoes are cooked through and the flavors have melded, remove the chili from heat.

8. Serve the vegetarian chili hot, garnished with optional toppings such as chopped fresh cilantro, diced avocado, shredded cheese, sour cream, and lime wedges. Enjoy the hearty and flavorful vegetarian chili with sweet potatoes and black beans!

This chili is packed with protein, fiber, and vitamins from the black beans and sweet potatoes, making it a nutritious and satisfying meal option. It's perfect for chilly evenings or for feeding a crowd at gatherings.

91. Baked salmon with pineapple salsa

Ingredients:
- 4 salmon fillets (about 6 ounces each), skin-on or skinless
- Salt and pepper to taste
- Olive oil
- 2 cups diced fresh pineapple
- 1/2 red onion, finely chopped
- 1 red bell pepper, diced
- 1 jalapeño pepper, seeded and finely chopped
- Juice of 1 lime
- 2 tablespoons chopped fresh cilantro
- Salt to taste

Instructions:
1. Preheat your oven to 400°F (200°C).

2. Season the salmon fillets with salt and pepper to taste. Drizzle with olive oil and rub to coat evenly.

3. Place the seasoned salmon fillets on a baking sheet lined with parchment paper or aluminum foil.

4. Bake in the preheated oven for about 12-15 minutes, or until the salmon is cooked through and flakes easily with a fork.

5. While the salmon is baking, prepare the pineapple salsa. In a mixing bowl, combine diced fresh pineapple, finely chopped red onion, diced red bell pepper, finely chopped jalapeño pepper, lime juice, chopped fresh cilantro, and salt to taste. Mix well to combine.

6. Once the salmon is cooked, remove it from the oven and let it rest for a few minutes.

7. Serve the baked salmon hot, topped with pineapple salsa.

8. Enjoy the delicious combination of tender baked salmon and sweet and tangy pineapple salsa!

This baked salmon with pineapple salsa is a light and flavorful dish that's perfect for a quick and healthy weeknight dinner. The juicy pineapple salsa adds a burst of freshness and color to the succulent salmon, making it a crowd-pleaser for any occasion.

92. Tuna and white bean salad

Ingredients:
- 2 cans (5 ounces each) of tuna, drained
- 1 can (15 ounces) of white beans (such as cannellini or Great Northern), drained and rinsed
- 1/2 red onion, finely chopped
- 1/2 cup diced cucumber
- 1/2 cup diced cherry tomatoes
- 2 tablespoons chopped fresh parsley
- Juice of 1 lemon
- 2 tablespoons extra virgin olive oil
- Salt and pepper to taste
- Optional: chopped fresh basil, olives, capers, or red pepper flakes for added flavor

Instructions:
1. In a large mixing bowl, combine drained tuna, white beans, finely chopped red onion, diced cucumber, diced cherry tomatoes, and chopped fresh parsley.

2. In a small bowl, whisk together the lemon juice and extra virgin olive oil to make the dressing.

3. Pour the dressing over the tuna and white bean mixture in the large bowl. Toss gently to coat everything evenly.

4. Season the salad with salt and pepper to taste. Adjust seasoning if necessary.

5. If desired, add optional ingredients such as chopped fresh basil, olives, capers, or red pepper flakes for extra flavor.
6. Once everything is well combined, chill the tuna and white bean sal
ad in the refrigerator for at least 30 minutes before serving to allow the flavors to meld.

7. Serve the chilled salad as is or over a bed of mixed greens.

8. Enjoy this flavorful and protein-packed tuna and white bean salad as a light and satisfying meal!

This salad is versatile and can be customized with your favorite ingredients. It's perfect for lunch, dinner, or as a side dish for picnics and gatherings. Feel free to experiment with different herbs, vegetables, and seasonings to suit your taste preferences.

93. Grilled chicken with mango and avocado salsa

Ingredients:
- 4 boneless, skinless chicken breasts
- Salt and pepper to taste
- Olive oil
- 2 ripe mangoes, diced
- 1 ripe avocado, diced
- 1/4 cup finely chopped red onion
- 1/4 cup chopped fresh cilantro
- Juice of 1 lime

Instructions:
1. Preheat grill to medium-high heat.

2. Season chicken breasts with salt and pepper, then drizzle with olive oil.

3. Grill chicken for about 6-8 minutes per side, until cooked through.

4. In a bowl, combine diced mangoes, avocado, red onion, cilantro, and lime juice to make salsa.

5. Serve grilled chicken topped with mango and avocado salsa.

Enjoy the vibrant flavors of grilled chicken with mango and avocado salsa!

94. Mediterranean chickpea salad

Ingredients:
- 2 cans (15 ounces each) chickpeas, drained and rinsed
- 1 English cucumber, diced
- 1 cup cherry tomatoes, halved
- 1/2 red onion, thinly sliced
- 1/4 cup chopped fresh parsley
- 1/4 cup chopped fresh mint
- 1/3 cup crumbled feta cheese
- Juice of 1 lemon
- 3 tablespoons extra virgin olive oil
- Salt and pepper to taste

Instructions:
1. In a large mixing bowl, combine chickpeas, diced cucumber, halved cherry tomatoes, thinly sliced red onion, chopped fresh parsley, and chopped fresh mint.

2. Crumble feta cheese over the salad ingredients.

3. In a small bowl, whisk together lemon juice, extra virgin olive oil, salt, and pepper to make the dressing.

4. Pour the dressing over the salad and toss gently to coat everything evenly.

5. Taste and adjust seasoning if necessary.

6. Serve the Mediterranean chickpea salad chilled or at room temperature.

Enjoy this refreshing and flavorful Mediterranean chickpea salad as a light meal or side dish!

95. Lentil and vegetable soup

Ingredients:
- 1 cup dried lentils, rinsed and drained
- 4 cups vegetable broth
- 1 onion, diced
- 2 carrots, diced
- 2 celery stalks, diced
- 2 cloves garlic, minced
- 1 can (14 ounces) diced tomatoes
- 2 teaspoons dried thyme
- 1 teaspoon dried oregano
- Salt and pepper to taste
- Olive oil for cooking
- Optional: chopped fresh parsley for garnish

Instructions:
1. In a large pot or Dutch oven, heat olive oil over medium heat.

2. Add diced onion, carrots, and celery to the pot. Cook until softened, about 5 minutes.

3. Add minced garlic to the pot and cook for another minute until fragrant.

4. Stir in dried lentils, vegetable broth, diced tomatoes (with their juices), dried thyme, and dried oregano.

5. Bring the soup to a boil, then reduce the heat to low. Cover and simmer for about 20-25 minutes, or until the lentils and vegetables are tender.

6. Once the soup is cooked, season with salt and pepper to taste. Adjust seasoning if necessary.

7. Serve the lentil and vegetable soup hot, garnished with chopped fresh parsley if desired.

Enjoy this hearty and nutritious lentil and vegetable soup as a comforting meal on a chilly day!

96. Grilled shrimp and vegetable skewers

Ingredients:
- 1 pound large shrimp, peeled and deveined
- 2 bell peppers (any color), cut into chunks
- 1 zucchini, sliced into rounds
- 1 red onion, cut into chunks
- Cherry tomatoes
- Olive oil
- Salt and pepper to taste
- Wooden or metal skewers

Marinade (optional):
- 3 tablespoons olive oil
- 2 cloves garlic, minced
- Juice of 1 lemon
- 1 teaspoon dried oregano
- 1 teaspoon paprika
- Salt and pepper to taste

Instructions:
1. If using wooden skewers, soak them in water for about 30 minutes to prevent burning.

2. In a bowl, whisk together the ingredients for the marinade, if using. Add the shrimp to the marinade and let it sit for about 15-20 minutes.

3. Preheat the grill to medium-high heat.

4. Thread the marinated shrimp onto skewers, alternating with chunks of bell peppers, zucchini slices, red onion chunks, and cherry tomatoes.

5. Brush the vegetable skewers with olive oil and season with salt and pepper.

6. Place the skewers on the preheated grill and cook for about 2-3 minutes per side, or until the shrimp is pink and opaque and the vegetables are tender and slightly charred.

7. Remove the skewers from the grill and serve immediately.

8. Enjoy these delicious grilled shrimp and vegetable skewers as a flavorful and healthy meal!

These grilled shrimp and vegetable skewers are perfect for summer barbecues or weeknight dinners. They're easy to make, customizable with your favorite vegetables, and packed with flavor!

97. Turkey and vegetable chili

Ingredients:
- 1 pound ground turkey
- 1 onion, diced
- 2 cloves garlic, minced
- 2 bell peppers (any color), diced
- 2 carrots, diced
- 2 celery stalks, diced
- 1 can (15 ounces) diced tomatoes
- 1 can (15 ounces) kidney beans, drained and rinsed
- 1 can (15 ounces) black beans, drained and rinsed
- 2 cups vegetable or chicken broth
- 2 tablespoons chili powder
- 1 teaspoon ground cumin
- 1 teaspoon paprika
- Salt and pepper to taste
- Olive oil for cooking
- Optional toppings: shredded cheese, chopped green onions, diced avocado, sour cream

Instructions:
1. In a large pot or Dutch oven, heat olive oil over medium heat.

2. Add diced onion, minced garlic, diced bell peppers, diced carrots, and diced celery to the pot. Cook until vegetables are softened, about 5-7 minutes.

3. Add ground turkey to the pot and cook until browned, breaking it up with a spoon as it cooks.

4. Stir in chili powder, ground cumin, paprika, salt, and pepper. Cook for another minute until fragrant.

5. Add diced tomatoes, kidney beans, black beans, and vegetable or chicken broth to the pot. Stir to combine.

6. Bring the chili to a boil, then reduce the heat to low. Cover and simmer for about 20-25 minutes, stirring occasionally.

7. Once the chili has thickened and the flavors have melded, taste and adjust seasoning if necessary. Serve the turkey and vegetable chili hot, garnished with your favorite toppings.

Enjoy this hearty and flavorful turkey and vegetable chili on a cold day or any time you're craving a comforting meal!

98. Spinach and feta stuffed tomatoes

Ingredients:
- 4 large tomatoes
- 2 cups fresh spinach, chopped
- 1/2 cup crumbled feta cheese
- 2 cloves garlic, minced
- 2 tablespoons olive oil
- Salt and pepper to taste
- Fresh basil leaves for garnish (optional)

Instructions:
1. Preheat your oven to 375°F (190°C).

2. Cut the tops off the tomatoes and scoop out the seeds and pulp with a spoon to create a hollow cavity. Place the hollowed-out tomatoes in a baking dish.

3. In a skillet, heat olive oil over medium heat. Add minced garlic and cook until fragrant, about 1 minute.

4. Add chopped spinach to the skillet and cook until wilted, about 2-3 minutes.

5. Remove the skillet from heat and stir in crumbled feta cheese. Season with salt and pepper to taste.

6. Spoon the spinach and feta mixture into the hollowed-out tomatoes, pressing gently to fill them evenly.

7. Place the stuffed tomatoes in the preheated oven and bake for about 20-25 minutes, or until the tomatoes are tender and the filling is heated through.

8. Once cooked, remove the stuffed tomatoes from the oven and let them cool for a few minutes. Garnish with fresh basil leaves if desired before serving.

Enjoy these delicious spinach and feta stuffed tomatoes as a flavorful and nutritious appetizer or side dish!

99. Baked cod with tomatoes and basil

Ingredients:
- 4 cod fillets (about 6 ounces each)
- Salt and pepper to taste
- 2 tablespoons olive oil
- 2 cloves garlic, minced
- 1 pint cherry tomatoes, halved
- 1/4 cup chopped fresh basil leaves
- Juice of 1 lemon
- Lemon wedges for serving
- Optional: grated Parmesan cheese for garnish

Instructions:
1. Preheat your oven to 400°F (200°C).

2. Season the cod fillets with salt and pepper to taste.

3. In a large oven-safe skillet or baking dish, heat olive oil over medium heat.

4. Add minced garlic to the skillet and cook for about 1 minute until fragrant.

5. Add cherry tomatoes to the skillet and cook for about 2-3 minutes until they start to soften.

6. Remove the skillet from heat and stir in chopped fresh basil.

7. Place the seasoned cod fillets on top of the tomato and basil mixture in the skillet.

8. Squeeze lemon juice over the cod fillets.

9. Transfer the skillet to the preheated oven and bake for about 15-20 minutes, or until the cod is cooked through and flakes easily with a fork.

10. Once cooked, remove the skillet from the oven.

11. Optionally, garnish the baked cod with grated Parmesan cheese before serving. Serve the baked cod with tomatoes and basil hot, with lemon wedges on the side.

100. Quinoa and roasted vegetable bowls

Ingredients:
- 1 cup quinoa, rinsed
- 2 cups water or vegetable broth
- 2 bell peppers (any color), sliced
- 1 zucchini, sliced
- 1 yellow squash, sliced
- 1 red onion, sliced
- 1 tablespoon olive oil
- Salt and pepper to taste
- Optional toppings: avocado slices, cherry tomatoes, fresh herbs, feta cheese, balsamic glaze

Instructions:
1. Preheat your oven to 400°F (200°C).

2. In a medium saucepan, bring water or vegetable broth to a boil. Add quinoa, reduce heat to low, cover, and simmer for about 15-20 minutes, or until quinoa is cooked and water is absorbed. Remove from heat and let it sit covered for 5 minutes, then fluff with a fork.

3. Meanwhile, spread sliced bell peppers, zucchini, yellow squash, and red onion on a baking sheet lined with parchment paper. Drizzle with olive oil and season with salt and pepper to taste. Toss to coat evenly.

4. Roast the vegetables in the preheated oven for about 20-25 minutes, or until tender and slightly caramelized, stirring halfway through cooking.

5. Divide cooked quinoa among serving bowls. Top with roasted vegetables.

6. Garnish with your choice of optional toppings, such as avocado slices, cherry tomatoes, fresh herbs, feta cheese, or a drizzle of balsamic glaze. Serve the quinoa and roasted vegetable bowls warm.

Enjoy these nutritious and flavorful quinoa and roasted vegetable bowls as a satisfying and wholesome meal!

As we conclude ***"Cookbook For Arthritis Weight Loss: Arthritis-Friendly Recipes for a Healthy Weight",*** we hope you feel empowered and inspired to take control of your health and well-being. This book has been crafted to provide you with the knowledge, tools, and delicious recipes needed to manage your weight effectively while living with arthritis.

Achieving and maintaining a healthy weight can significantly alleviate arthritis symptoms, reduce inflammation, and improve your overall quality of life. By integrating the nutrient-rich, anti-inflammatory recipes from this book into your daily routine, you are making a proactive choice to support your joint health and enhance your vitality.

Remember, the journey to better health is unique for everyone. It's essential to be patient with yourself and celebrate each small victory along the way. Sustainable weight loss is about making gradual, consistent changes that become part of your lifestyle. Focus on the progress you've made, rather than striving for perfection.

In addition to the recipes, the practical tips and strategies provided in this book are designed to help you navigate the challenges of weight management with arthritis. From mindful eating and portion control to low-impact exercises and stress management techniques, we've covered a holistic approach to support your journey.

As you continue on this path, keep exploring new recipes and finding joy in cooking and eating nutritious meals. The more you enjoy the process, the easier it will be to maintain these healthy habits long-term. Your commitment to a healthier lifestyle not only benefits your joints but also contributes to your overall well-being and happiness.

We hope that this book has been a valuable resource for you and that it will continue to serve as a guide and inspiration for your health journey. Your dedication to improving your health is commendable, and we are honored to have been a part of it.

Thank you for choosing "Cookbook For Arthritis Weight Loss: Arthritis-Friendly Recipes for a Healthy Weight." May your days be filled with delicious meals, reduced pain, and a renewed sense of well-being.

Warm regards,

Author of "Cookbook For Arthritis Weight Loss: Arthritis-Friendly Recipes for a Healthy Weight"